The strange story of False Hair

By the same author

The Strange Story of False Teeth
The Truth about Cottages
The Story of the Bicycle

The strange story of **False Hair**

by

John Woodforde

Routledge & Kegan Paul
London

First published 1971
by Routledge & Kegan Paul Ltd
Broadway House, 68–74 Carter Lane
London EC4V 5EL
Photoset in Great Britain by BAS Printers Limited,
Wallop, Hampshire. Set in Plantin 110

ISBN 0 7100 7095 0

To Sue

Contents

Illustrations

Acknowledgment

I have made several references in the text to the work of Mr James Stevens Cox, hairdresser, wigmaker, publisher and antiquarian bookseller, and especially to his *Dictionary of Hairdressing and Wigmaking* published in 1966 by the Hairdressers' Technical Council, but I would like here to express gratitude for typescript-reading and kindly advice.

One

Wigs galore

'One lock of hair falling across the temples', observed William Hogarth, surveying the English head in 1753, 'has an effect too alluring to be strictly decent.' The significance of the head is so great that the least adjustment to its decoration, such as tilting a hat an inch to the side, will govern the impression a person creates. A wig can alter him almost beyond recognition.

Wigs have always been a subject for serious thought. In the eighteenth century the wigs worn by men indicated status, social class and beliefs, and were taken so seriously that a good barber would offer a choice of twenty or thirty styles. Today, too, there are numerous types of wig on offer. Only some of the people who wear them are bald. In the big stores and, of course, in the hairdressing establishments, wigs of fashion—or convenience—are being bought by men with healthy hair of their own, but hair which they think unsuitable for a particular occasion. It has even been possible, since 1970, to hire men's wigs for an evening from clothes hire firms.

Instant length is the main draw for these wigs. And hair as long as a girl's need not today suggest that a man is decadent. People are prepared to concede, as they did in the seventeenth century just before the start of the great wig era (when Cromwell himself had hair to his shoulders), that there is nothing axiomatic about the correctness of the short haircut. Long hair—source of wigmakers' profits—was the secret of the strength of Samson; it was the legitimate pride of the ancient Parthians, the Persians, the Lacedaemonian

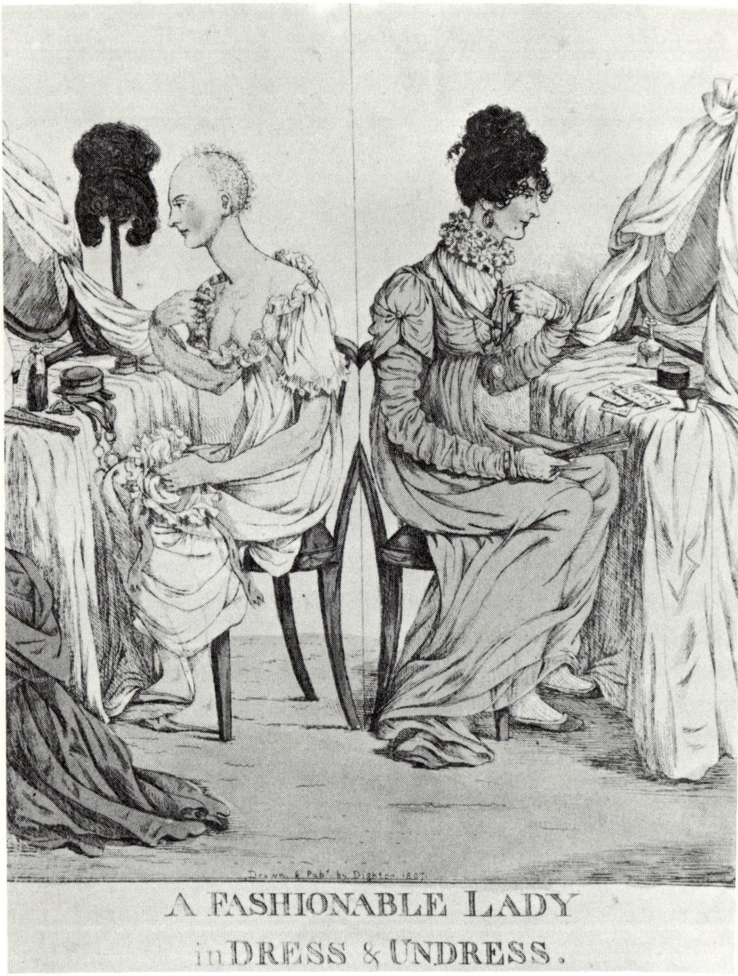

A print of 1807 after Robert Dighton

infantry and the Athenian cavalry. Homer wrote of 'long haired' Greeks to signify an honourable distinction. The Goths regarded mown-down hair as a mark of thraldom. According to Pliny, the extremely long hair of the Gauls led to the region where they lived being referred to as *Gallia comata*, hairy Gaul; Julius Caesar made conquered Gauls cut off their hair as a token of submission. Not surprisingly, length of hair was the prime consideration in the construction of the first European wigs for men; these contained hair which was longer and fuller than any one scalp could grow.

Women's preoccupation with fashion wigs has usually, throughout history, had to do with pretending they were not wigs, with fear of exposure and of being thought deceitful.* A new attitude to false hair came in with the craze of the 1960s for slip-on hairdos for an evening out. It was a craze which spread so fast that now about a third of the women of Britain and the United States possess a time-saving wig of convenience. In offices and shops girls try out one another's machine-made wigs of glossy Asian hair or nylon. In private life a housewife entertaining need not abandon her intention of popping on a wig if an early guest discovers her without it.

One result of good trade in frivolous wigs, and of the way they are now cheerfully spoken of, is that people worried by baldness have grown readier to seek a wigmaker. The subject has shed much of its embarrassment. Did not a hairdresser claim recently in a newspaper interview: 'A few wigs are becoming an essential part of the well-dressed man's wardrobe'?

The wigmakers for their part believe they have polished up some of their techniques in the last ten years; they have certainly tried many experiments, improved their advertising and made their products more easily available. In 1960 the classified commercial section of the New York tele-

* Some orthodox Jewish brides, on the other hand, still guarantee their vows of fidelity by cropping their hair and wearing a rather obvious wig

phone directory had only two or three pages devoted to hair goods. In 1970 it had thirteen such pages, from A.A.A. Wig Corporation to Leo Zucker Industries. Whole new industries have grown up to provide wig straps and adhesives, wig stands, wig cases, display turntables and display heads. New terms have been created and old terms revived: cascades, chignons, falls, dome falls. There is always, as evidence of use, a large quantity of false hair awaiting collection in the lost property offices of the railways and airlines.

The term false hair, used several times in these pages, is obviously inaccurate when it refers to material which once grew naturally, but it is a term which has been found convenient for centuries as an alternative to the professional's *postiche* (the French for sham), covering all hairpieces from wigs to pincurls. The word wig, generally denoting a full head of bought hair, dates from about 1675; it was derived from the French *perruque* (itself derived from the Italian *perruca*) following a run in English through such forms as peruke, periwyk and periwig—or periwigg as spelled by Pepys and Lyly: in *Euphues*, 1579, Lyly pleasantly wrote it perywigge. The shortened form, wig, first came into use in the 1670s.

Little has been published in English about the technique of making wigs; British and American wigmakers have always had secrets to guard, today no less than in former times. Denis Diderot in his *Encyclopédie* and Garsault in *Art du perruquier* recorded contemporarily the techniques of the mid-eighteenth century wigmakers in France, but the first comparable work in English was Edwin Creer's *Boardwork or the Art of Wigmaking*, 1887. Since that date there has appeared only one book devoted entirely to the details of wigmaking. This book, spilling at least most of the beans, is *Manual of Wigmaking*, written in a pleasant and lucid manner by Mary Botham and Leslie Sharrad and published in 1964. It is not surprising, in the present wig-conscious period, to find that the book has been reprinted again and again.

Two

Ancient Egyptian and Roman wigs

The ancient Egyptians made use of wigs, and a number of them survive still in museums; there is one at the British Museum in London. They were highly stylized wigs and worn mainly, it seems, on formal or festive occasions; they can rarely have been used to hide natural defects since it was a common Egyptian practice to make the head bald artificially by shaving it.

The late Dr Margaret Murray believed that wigs originated in Egypt, and in *The Splendour that was Egypt*, 1949, she put forward the theory that wearing them was at first a royal prerogative; that the pharaoh, when appearing in public, did not wish his subjects to see the sacred head naked.

From at least 3000 B.C., so it appears from ancient paintings, both men and women of high rank wore wigs with 'full dress'. They were made from human hair—sometimes from vegetable fibre or grass—and would consist of neatly

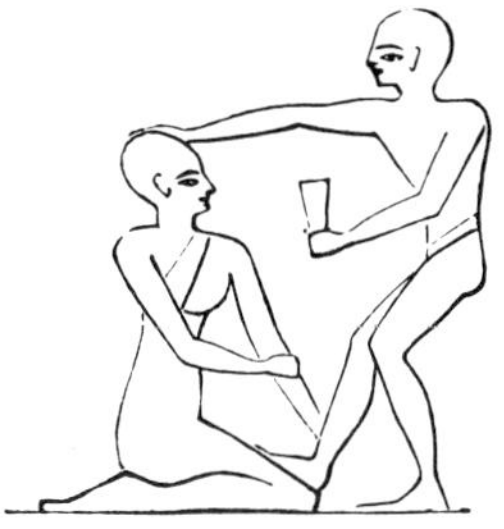

Shaven Egyptian heads

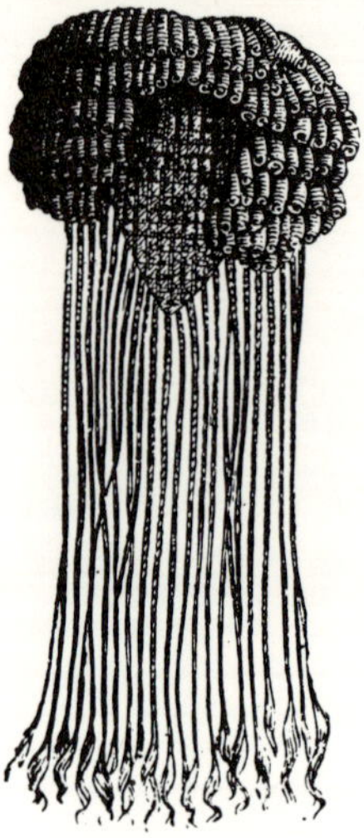

Ancient Egyptian wig similar to a specimen in the British Museum

formed plaits and braids. Around 1000 B.C. they became large enough to give the wearer a top-heavy appearance. Queen Isimkheb, who lived approximately 900 years before Christ, had a vast wig with a mass of small curls and with dozens of long narrow plaits behind.

This wig was one of fifteen in the Cairo Museum analysed chemically and microscopically in 1930 by Alfred Lucas, author of *Ancient Egyptian Materials and Industries*, 1934.

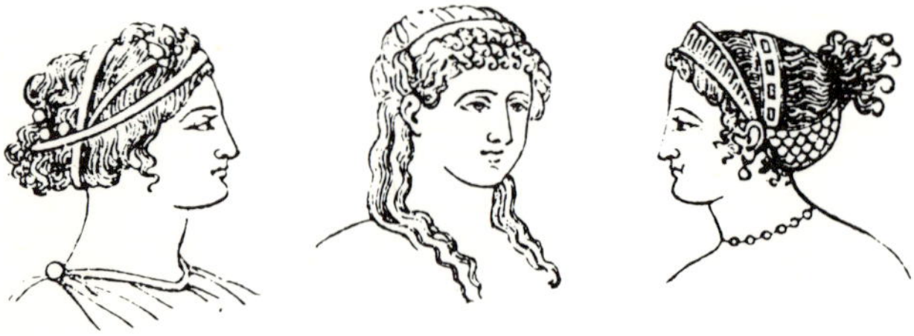

Greek women with strophos head-dress and, far right, nimbo head-dress

It was black and had been officially described as made of hair mixed with the wool of a black sheep. Mr Lucas discovered that both this wig and twelve of the rest consisted of brown human hair only. There were two wigs of Roman date, of which one was made from date palm fibre and the other grass. To hold the hairdressing work in position, all the hair wigs had been treated with a wax which was identified by its melting point and other properties as beeswax.

Wigs were certainly known in other early civilizations, the Mesopotamian, for example; stage wigs were an accepted convention in the theatre of ancient Greece.

Later on, among Roman women, wigs became extremely fashionable. They offered an easy way of seeming blonde, a state considered desirable in a land of dark heads. Numerous wigs were made with fine flaxen hair collected from the conquered Germanic natives of Northern Europe. In the first century Ovid writes, in *Ars Amatoria*, that a woman friend whose hair is falling out through illness will find there is still plenty of German hair to be had.

Hair that was dyed yellow was associated with women engaged in prostitution. Messalina, the strange nymphomaniac wife of Claudius I, used to put on a yellow wig (Juvenal offers chapter and verse for this) for visiting Roman brothels.

The female wigs of Rome would not have looked life-like to modern eyes; but nor would the natural hair, so rigid was

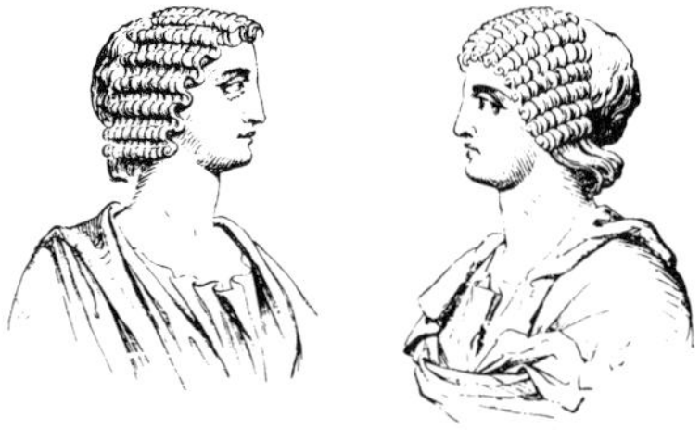

Roman women in what are thought to be wigs.
Drawings from statuary

the manner of crimping it. Much effort was expended on this crimping and on the finishing-off with ribbons, flowers and jewellery: yet the basic arrangement was simple for most of the Roman period—a central parting with a knot of hair either on top or at the back.

Wigs were worn by Roman men, too, but generally only by those who wanted to hide a defect of nature. They would be reticent about it, and would not order an unlikely colour like flaxen.

To judge by the workmanship of the Roman wigs which are still to be seen in museums, it was quite possible for a man's necessity wig to look life-like. There was no need for the wigmakers to simulate either a parting or a hair line—both very difficult—since it was customary for all men's hair to be combed forward and hang, like Julius Caesar's, in tapers on the forehead. The deception could indeed have been clever enough to be embarrassing when exposed. Flavius Avianus, a second-century poet, writes in *Fabulae* of the distress of a bald knight when his wig blew off while he was riding.

The poet Martial was deadly in his *Epigrams*—in a rather pointless way—about men who tried to improve their appearance with wigs. He refers, for example, to an acquaintance called Lentinus, who has taken the trouble to exchange thinning hair for a black wig, and says that his wig would deceive no one even if it was secure (apparently it

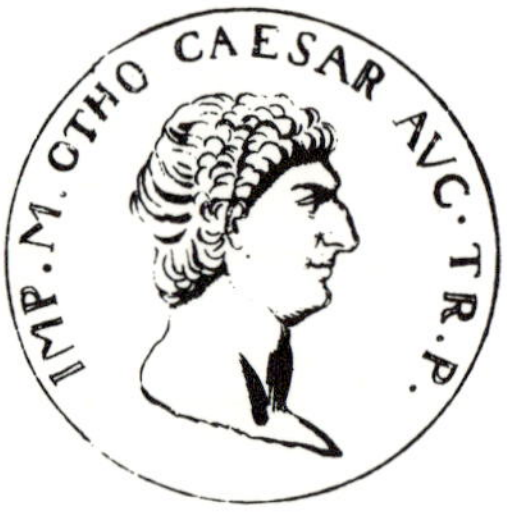

Otho, Roman Emperor, A.D. 69. He wore a wig all the time to conceal baldness

once fell off); he impertinently warns another acquaintance that, for aping youth, the Queen of thc Shades will pluck the mask from his head.

Martial was even more scornful, indeed cruel, in lines addressed to women of easy virtue allegedly seeking to win attraction by dishonest means. 'You use, Laelia, and are not ashamed, teeth and hair that you have bought. But what will you do for an eye?' Propertius also wrote with disdain of girls and women who bought hair. Like Martial, he was loose in his love life but rigid in condemning the false curl.

As an alternative to a wig, some bald men actually had hair painted on their skulls. Martial wrote to one such man: 'You fob us off with fictitious hair—your dirty bald scalp is covered with locks represented in paint. You have no occasion for a barber for your head; you may shave yourself much better, Phoebus, with a sponge.'

Phoebus apparently took notice and gave up painting his head, for Martial has this to say in a subsequent epigram: 'As you cover with a kid's skin your temples and the crown of your bald pate, he made a happy remark to you, Phoebus, who told you that your head was well shod.'

The wearing of skin skull-caps seems to have been fairly common among men who were bald or who worked all day in the open; they always had the fur outside. The *Dictionnaire François-Celtique* of 1732[2] refers to a cap of this sort being still worn in Brittany; it is described as 'a poor man's

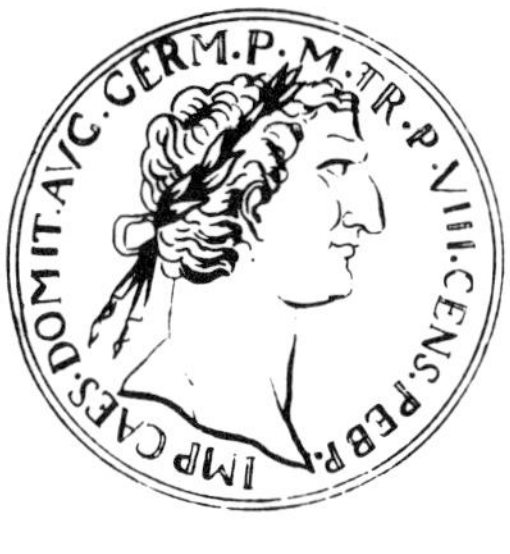

Domitian, Roman Emperor, *c.* A.D. 95. He was totally bald, but his coins and medals show him otherwise

peruke made of sheepskin with the wool uppermost'.

It is known from the records of contemporaries and early historians that wigs had a place, for various reasons, in the wardrobes of several of the Roman emperors. Caligula is said to have put on a wig to disguise himself while prowling at night in search of pleasure. Caracalla, according to Herodian, sought to ingratiate himself, on visiting a Danube-side settlement, by wearing not only German dress but also a blonde wig trimmed in the local style.* Plutarch wrote of wigs being worn by Hadrian and Otho: the latter kept a wig on all the time, anxious for it not to be seen that he was bald.

Some of the wigs of great Romans would have been no more than hat-like adornments to be slipped on and off at whim. How much they were used in this way is a matter for guesswork. But it is by no means incredible to read in Evelyn Waugh's historical novel *Helena*, 1950, that the Emperor Constantine received his mother at the Palatine in a small green wig. 'My dear boy, what have you got on your head?' . . . 'Don't you like it?' he asked anxiously. 'Do you think it makes me look pale?'

* Caracalla's everyday hair-style, as depicted on his coins, was the inspiration for a ladies' fashion wig of 1790 featuring curls that resembled sausages

Three

Modesty and the hair

The early Christian Church tried to stamp out the wearing of wigs, especially among women. To the early Fathers embellishment of the head with false hair was an affront to chastity, an enticement to illicit pleasures. No doubt their suspicions were often justified. Clement of Alexandria in the first century A.D. liked to declare that it was impossible for anyone in a wig to receive a priest's blessing offered by the laying on of hands: the benediction could not pass through the hair of a stranger. Tertullian in the second century said that all personal disguise was adulterous. 'All wigs are such disguises and inventions of the devil . . . if you will not throw away your false hair as hateful to Heaven, let me make it hateful to you by reminding you that it may well have come from the head of a damned person or an unclean person.' Cyprian in the third century drew attention to the wearing of veils by 'the pagans'. 'What better are you than pagans if you come to prayers in wigs?'

Clearly women wore their false hair in a way that was both alluring and detectable by the clergy. For century after century the councils of the Church of Rome condemned its use. In A.D. 692 the Council of Constantinople actually excommunicated a number of wig-wearing Christians. Some local synods would authorize no hair-style which was not short and straight; the priests themselves trimmed their hair under threat of forfeiture of revenues or benefice.

By the twelfth century, women were avoiding thunderous accusations of immodesty by wearing, in public at least, a decorous and often charming fabric head-dress. Men, on the other hand, would be reproved for having their hair too long—usually it was their own hair, though the use of male wigs was not unknown. St Anselm (d.1109), Archbishop of Canterbury, was uncompromising about men with long hair. His biographer, Eadmer, reports that he once put several aristocratic young men on penance and refused them absolution until they had agreed to be close shorn. St Anslem would allow no one with long hair, natural or false, in his cathedral.

King Henry I (d.1135), though allowed few marks in modern history books for moral rectitude, features in Camden's *Remains Concerning Britain*, 1623, as a king who 'reprehended immodesty of apparel . . . and abolished the wearing of long hair with locks and perukes'. There may be a bearing on this unlikely statement in another anecdote about Henry to the effect that the length of his own hair was so much criticized by the Bishop of Séez, during a visit to Normandy, that he had it cut short on the spot. French kings, who had traditionally enjoyed the privilege of having hair as long as they liked under the 'droit de chevelure royale', were now falling in with the wishes of the Church and wore hair that was cut short. It was not until the seventeenth century that the Church's influence on hair-styles ceased to be effective.

The women of England and France continued to conceal their hair, often under a gable-shaped hood, until the middle of the sixteenth century. Around the year 1540 hoods got smaller and rather more hair was allowed to show. One thing led to another and, after 1580, the hair rather than the hood became the chief ornament of the head. It was now the fashion to arrange it in masses of small curls; it even became acceptable for the hair in front to be built up slightly over pads and wire frames. However, the arrangement as a whole was confined and symmetrical.

Here and there great ladies found it pleasanter to keep an array of wigs than to sit through regular treatments necessary for maintaining numerous small curls. And thus began, among women, the first English vogue for the wig of fashion. If any one person can be said to have started the vogue, it was Queen Elizabeth I who possessed, in later life, a large number of neatly curled wigs. For her, there was an unsightly deficiency which had to be hidden; but many of the ladies of her court, whatever the condition of their own hair, hastened to follow her example. Those who did not wear a wig at least showed their respect for the Queen by having their hair dyed one or other of the Queen's favourite colours, auburn and saffron yellow.

There was nothing flaunting or immodest about these late-sixteenth-century wigs for women. Moreover, they imitated the natural hair closely enough to stifle any reproaches a stern moralist might have had in mind to make. The fact that Mary Queen of Scots wore a wig (she kept an array of auburn wigs) was unknown even by people well acquainted with her; indeed, at the time of her death many learned with feelings of shock that her attractive auburn hair was not her own. A type of lace-edged head-dress which she liked to wear dipping to a point above the forehead became known as Mary Stuart head-dresses; wigs, too, were formed with a Mary Stuart central peak.

Four

The royal and clerical wigs of France

Henry III of France set a precedent by growing his hair as long as he could, but quite early in life he lost it all as a result of dyeing it with untried chemicals. Thereafter he always wore either a kind of turban or a velvet cap with tufts of hair sewn just beneath the brim.

His courtiers had followed his example in taking to long hair, and now some of them copied his hair-fringed caps. 'Those pretty pets of the Court,' wrote Pierre de l'Estoile in his memoirs, 'what pains they took over the curling and re-curling of their long hair.' Montaigne said they were all effeminate. It was under Henry III, King of France from

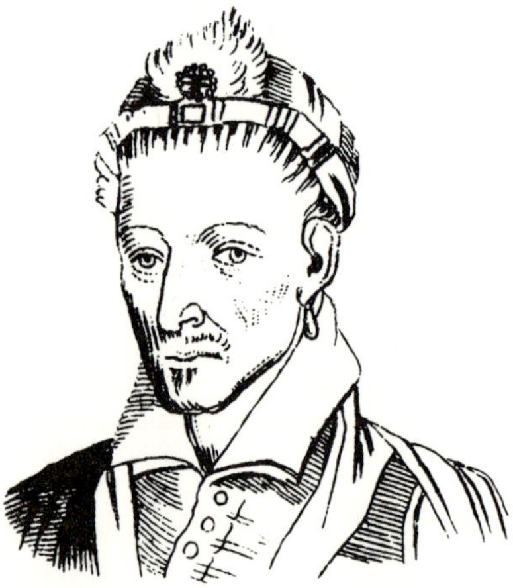

Henry III of France, *c.* 1580, wearing a cap to which a fringe of false hair has been attached

1574 to 1589 (and described in history books as ill-favoured and vain), that false hair first came to be used in French court circles.

In 1620 Abbé de la Rivière appeared at the court of Louis XIII in a full wig of blonde hair. It was a great success. Four years later the king himself adopted a wig, initiating a fashion which was in due course to spread throughout Europe. From the natural appearance of the wig, as depicted in Louis' portraits, it would seem that the art of wig-making was already well advanced. Certainly the wig-makers of Paris were busy experimenting, especially with ways of attaching hairs to a caul, but the men's wigs of this time are said to have overheated the head and to have caused a scratching sound at the ears. They were also unstable.

The great King Louis XIV was responsible, despite himself, for the final triumph of the wig as an accepted item of male attire; as a young man he was happy with his own abundant hair and scorned wig-wearing, but the start of baldness at thirty-two made him change his mind. His long wigs were voluminous, majestic and black: only in extreme

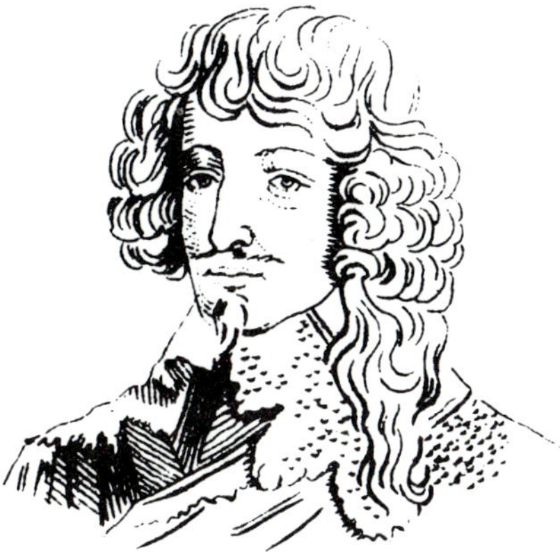

Louis XIII of France, *c.* 1625. The asymmetrical design of his wig was taken up in England in the latter years of the seventeenth century; it was always the left-hand side which was the longer

age would he permit a light sprinkling of powder to suggest a becoming greyness. M. Binet, his barber, used to boast that he would crop the heads of any number of Frenchmen to ensure that the king's head remained properly covered.

Binet designed some very handsome wigs, one of which, dating from 1680, was known as 'devant à la Fontange' after a favourite mistress of the king.[3] Such was Binet's fame that *binette* became a jocular French word for a head. It is still in colloquial use but now means a face, as in 'quelle binette!' 'what a face!'

Louis XIV seems to have retained a certain diffidence about the nakedness of his head beneath the wig and Binet, according to the researches of Mr Turner Wilcox,[4] was the only person ever to see him *sans perruque*. When he retired at night, the king handed out his wig to a page through drawn bed curtains; and in the morning, when the wig had to be returned to him, it was again passed through drawn curtains. With his successor Louis XV, who kept plenty of his own hair (in stubble form), the morning procedure was different: 'The Lord Chamberlain or the First Lord of the Bedchamber removes the king's nightcap, and one of the barbers combs the king's hair, at which point begins the *première entrée*, that is to say, the page admits those who have the right to enter in virtue of their office . . . when the king's hair has been sufficiently combed, M. Quentin [the chief barber] hands him the wig he uses while dressing, which is shorter than the one he usually wears for the rest of the day . . .'[5]

By 1634 forty barber-wigmakers had appointments to serve the Court at Versailles. In 1673 Louis XIV created a new guild of 200 barber-wigmakers for the City of Paris, a number he increased in 1691 to 300.* As well as being the only people with official permission to dress hair for gain, the barber-wigmakers had the right to preside over hot bath houses. Payments for licences provided an acceptable revenue for the royal treasury; but Colbert, Louis' finance

* By the year 1760 the number had risen to 850

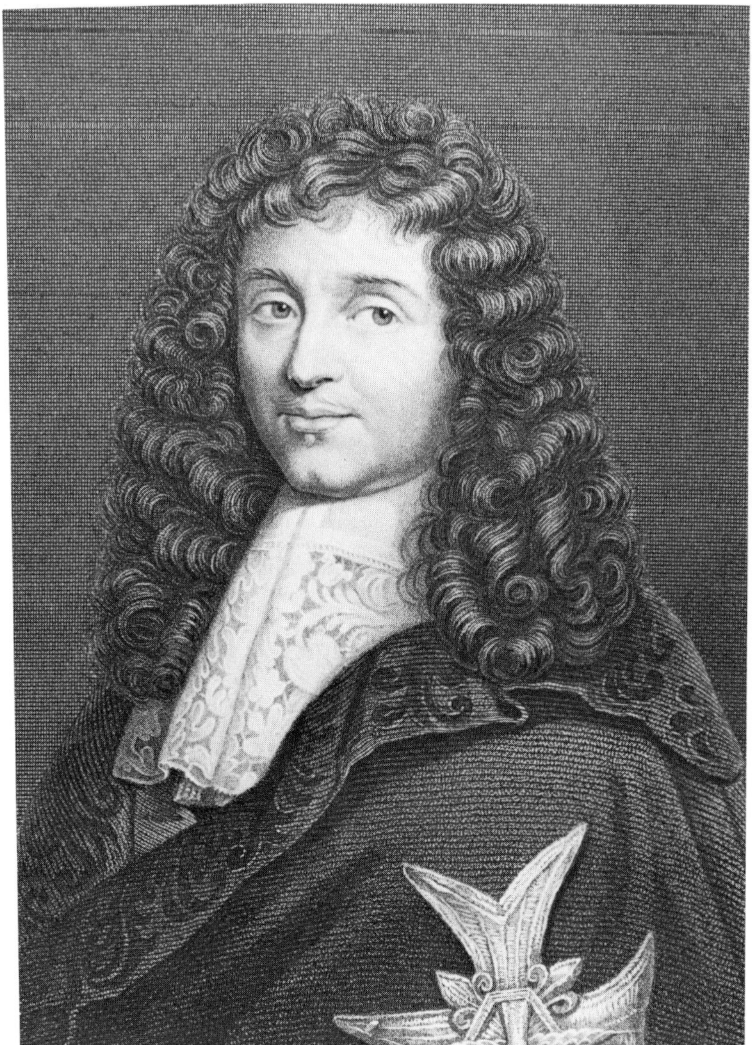

Jean Baptiste Colbert, *c.* 1660 in a typical French full wig minister, deplored the amount of money that was being spent outside France on the purchase of hair, and threatened to put an end to these imports. The wigmakers had no difficulty in demonstrating that, since they were almost the sole suppliers of finished wigs to neighbouring countries—where the use of them was spreading—they caused a greater amount of money to enter France than the amount leaving for the purchase of hair.

Despite the hostility of the synods and councils of the Church and the threats of excommunication, there were plenty of priests who wore the fashionable long curling wig. The matter of wigs split the Church, both that of Rome and the Reformed Church: as more and more priests took to them, the indignation of strict churchmen became extreme. The Bishop of Toul issued a statement saying that the fashion unchristianized any who adopted it; a man had better not pray at all than pray with his head bewigged.

In 1690 Jean-Baptiste Thiers, parish priest of Champrond, published at his own expense a book of 550 pages about wigs and the clergy. Despite a laconic title, *Histoire des perruques*, the book's main purpose was to expose current practices which Dr Thiers considered monstrous and wicked. There are stories of priests spending such and such a sum annually at their barbers, of priests who kept their best wigs for the drawing-room and wore inferior wigs in church, of priests turned out of their livings for wearing wigs—only to be welcomed by the easy-going bishop of another diocese. Acrimonious scenes took place in vestries, apparently, between wigged priests preparing themselves for the altar and other priests trying to knock their wigs off. Dr Thiers supported his remarks by so many quotations from speakers at Church councils and synods that his repetitious book became a Bible for all who wanted to attack wig-wearing.

The Archbishop of Reims believed he had settled the dispute within the Church by decreeing that in certain circumstances wigs might be worn: they were permitted, though not at the actual altar, for priests who were infirm or of great age. One result was that a priest might keep on his wig until he was within feet of the altar and then take it off and hand it to an assistant.

The clergy in England rarely wore wigs until they became the general fashion in the 1660s. Possibly it was because they regretted not doing so that they sometimes reproved members of their congregations for having hair they thought unduly long. Around 1690, when Dr Thiers' attack on wig-wearing came out, Archbishop Tillotson (wearing his bishop's wig) was able to recall in a sermon the days when 'ministers, whatever their text, did either find or make occasion to reprove the great sin of long hair; and if they saw anyone in the congregation guilty in that way, they would point him out and let fly at him'.[6]

Five

Periwigs of the Restoration period

The Frenchman's fashion of wearing a wig over perfectly good natural hair was ignored in England until the second half of the seventeenth century. Even the totally bald might prefer to sew bunches of hair round the rim of a hat:[7] hats with brims were worn indoors and outdoors on all but the least formal occasions and always at meals.* Periwigs, it was agreed, belonged to the theatre, to entertainers like Shakespeare's 'rumbustious periwig-pated fellow tearing a passion to tatters'.

All the same, men began to take more interest, after about 1610, in the ornamental possibilities of hair. Under Queen Elizabeth it had been combed straight back and kept above the ears. Now, though still combed back, it was allowed to grow—and the disappearance of high ruffs in favour of flat collars gave it plenty of room. In the 1620s it was not uncommon for a man's hair to fall in ringlets to his lace-edged collar. And it was fashionable to follow James I in cultivating a love lock. This was a single bunch of hair, longer than all the rest, which was brought forward from the nape of the neck, tied at the tip with a ribbon and disposed casually on the chest.

After 1630 it was usual for hair to reach the shoulders and back; a fringe at the forehead was brushed to one side. With elaborate clothes of velvet and lace, with feathers and ribbons, most men made their women look sombre. There were even plenty of so-called Roundheads, including

* Samuel Pepys in a diary entry for 1664 blames a cold in the head on not wearing his hat at dinner

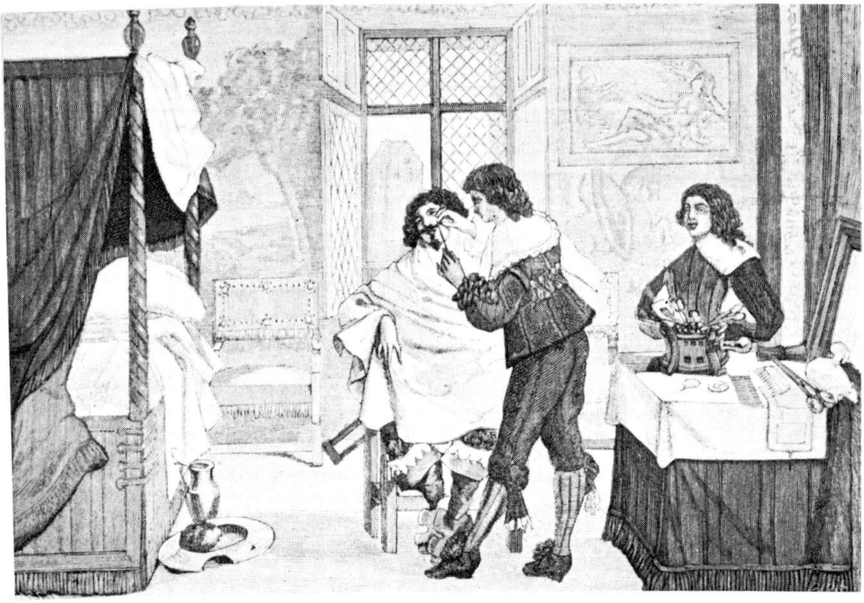

French barber, and assistant, grooming a customer in his bedroom

Cromwell himself, whose hair flowed far below the ears.

Concerned as they were with a flattering frame for the face, Englishmen were ready for the wig-wearing fashion which came with the Restoration of the Monarchy in 1660, when Charles II and his followers returned from exile on the Continent.

The large French wigs worn at Court, and rapidly copied elsewhere, had the flamboyance of other Restoration objects. They can even be compared, for example, with the floridly-carved highback chairs. Like the stretchers and uprights of these, the long dangling locks of hair were formed in barley sugar twists; and both the backs of the chairs and the crowns of the wigs were surmounted with crest forms.

Despite their grandeur, Restoration fashion wigs—black or brown, and unpowdered—imitated natural hair more closely than those which emerged in the eighteenth century.

They came to be known as full-bottom wigs to distinguish them from the bobbed wigs later adopted by tradesmen. A version of the full-bottom called the travelling wig had the hair gathered into two great twists which could be tied back in a queue.

The large wigs were relatively heavy to wear but at least, when they were taken off, the shaved head felt pleasantly light and could be readily washed and dried. Although considerations of hygiene had nothing to do with the start of the fashion, they were certainly a factor in keeping it going. With the soaps available, the cleaning of shoulder-length hair was difficult, the removal of clinging lice-nits impossible. With a shaved head and a wig—preferably several wigs—the scalp need never itch for long; nor need hairdressing take place on the head. In a play of 1673 a character is reminded of the old days when, instead of a periwig, he wore his own 'slink, greasy hair'.[8]

Wigs had their uses, too, as a cloak for the identity. Just how far a new head of hair can alter a man was being demonstrated by the way guileless acquaintances would fail to recognize one another in the street. The materials were ready to hand for those with reason to go incognito. 'For vailing of their visages,' wrote Sir Henry Wotton of two such people, 'his highness and the marquis bought each a perriwig somewhat to overshadow their foreheads.'

Samuel Pepys, who became an eminent civil servant, offers in his diaries the best account of what it was like for a young man to be confronted with the fashion for full-bottom wigs. Pepys was anxious to fit himself for mixing with the eminent, yet he was barely thirty and had luxuriant hair of his own. His barber, Jervas, keeps on trying to persuade him to have it cut off and one day invites him to try the effect of false hair. 'I did try', Pepys writes, 'two or three borders and periwigs, meaning to wear one; and yet I have no stomach for it; but that the pains of keeping my own hair clean is so great.' He also speculates on 'the trouble that I foresee will be in wearing them'.

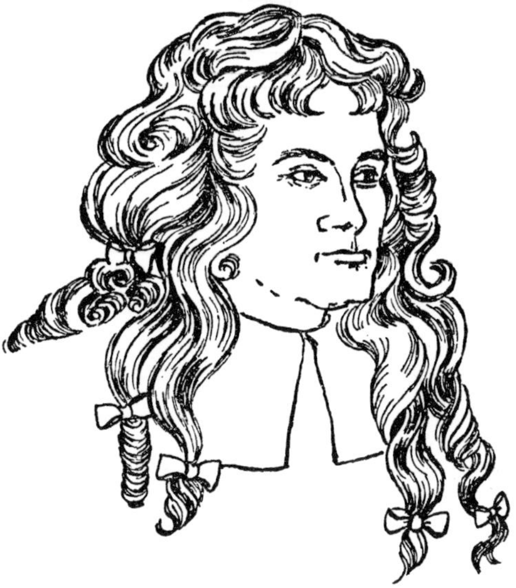

Restoration wigs at first imitated the natural hair

At length he succumbs, and towards the end of 1663 submits himself for the hair-cutting ordeal. 'It went a little to my heart to part with it at present, but it being over and my periwig on, I paid him [Jervas] £3 for it; and away went he with my own hair to make up another of.'

He is diffident to start with, and grateful for the admiring comments of his wife and maid servants. However, going to church in the wig for the first time 'did not prove so strange as I was afraid it would'. It is not necessary to turn many pages in his diary to find him well satisfied with his changed appearance and happily choosing a better wig box.

In April 1665 Pepys is briefly wigless again, having sent his wig to Jervas for cleaning and repairs. He writes that 'having suffered my own hair to grow long, in order to wear it, I find the convenience of periwigs is so great, that I have cut off all short again and will keep to periwigs'.

Later on he becomes rather worried about the origin of

the bought hair. He records on a Sunday in September 1665: 'Up, and put on my coloured silk suit, very fine, and my new periwig, bought a good while since, but durst not wear, because the plague was in Westminster when I bought it; and it is a wonder what will be the fashion, after the plague is done, as to periwigs, for nobody will dare to buy any hair for fear of the infection, that it had been cut off the heads of people dead of the plague.'

Nevertheless the following year Pepys bought two wigs at once. They were expensive at £4 10s the pair. He described them as 'mighty fine; indeed too fine, I thought, for me'. One of them 'made a great show' in church.

Seventeenth-century household accounts reveal to what a large extent the fashion for wigs augmented expenditure on apparel. In 1672 the Earl of Bedford's bill from the Woburn wigmaker came to £54 10s. He had four new wigs in the year, ranging in price from £6 to £20; one at £10 was described as 'a periwig for riding'.[9]

Under James II wigs became vast, each requiring the growth from several heads. They had two great horns of hair rising up in front on each side of a parting and gave rise to the term 'bigwig' for a wealthy or important person. The fine gentlemen beneath them had no diffidence about adjusting curls ruffled by slumber or dalliance with women. They carried combs in their ample pockets (pockets in clothes were an invention of the seventeenth century) and used them openly in coffee houses and theatres. Dryden, in *Almanzer and Almahide*, 1670, makes a reference to the smart theatregoer 'managing his comb with grace'.

In the 1680s men began to give up wearing hats indoors, even in church. Hats tended to spoil the top part of a wig. By the 1690s wigs had become too cumbersome to be single-piece articles and came in three parts, one to hang down the back and the other two to hang in front upon the shoulders. Some men had wigs that reached almost to the waist, the left-hand side usually a few inches longer than the right. Large wigs were associated—only half in jest—with good

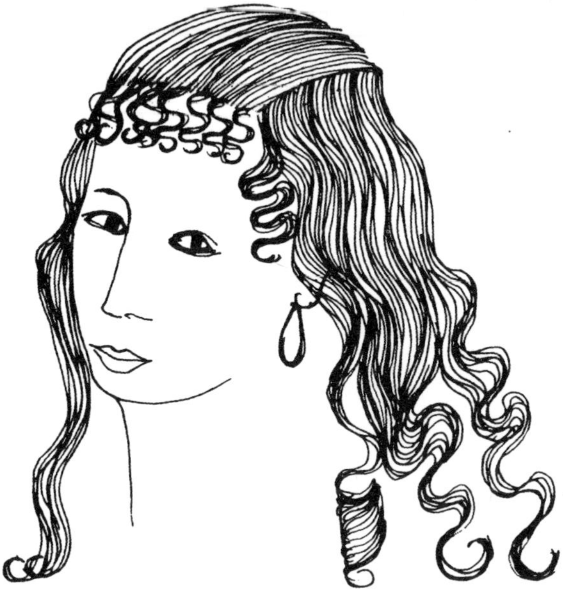

High forehead decorated with thin wisps of curl, *c.* 1660

minds. 'A full wig', says a character in George Farquhar's *Love in a Bottle*, 1699, 'is as infallible a token of wit as the laurel.'

Women, during most of the seventeenth century, allowed their hair to look rather like the men's. Conventions about one style being feminine and another masculine barely existed. When men took to hanging side locks, so did women; and in the latter part of the century, both sexes arranged their hair, natural or false, in twin peaks on the top of the head. But a fashion peculiar to women, inspired by Italy, was to acquire by plucking a high dome-like forehead, and to decorate it with thin, wispy curls. This rudimentary fringe sprang from a transverse parting; behind it the hair was strained back to form a bun.

Full wigs for women were unusual except with riding clothes; a very correct, and very masculine, riding wig had long dark curls and ringlets which covered the shoulders (some Cavaliers' wives and daughters wore their own hair like this). There is a record[10] of Lady Grisell Baillie paying in 1690 the large sum of £28 for a long riding wig.

It was not only in their hair arrangements that men and women looked alike. Pepys writes in 1666: 'Walking in the galleries at Whitehall, I find the ladies of honour dressed in their riding-garbs, with coats and doublets with deep skirts just for all the world like mine . . . and with periwigs and with hats. So that only for a long petticoat dragging under their men's coats, nobody could take them for women in any point whatever; which was an odd sight and a sight which did not please me.'

Six

Full-bottoms, tyes, bags and bobs

By the beginning of the eighteenth century even villages would have a barber with a knowledge of wigmaking; it had become so much the male custom to wear a wig that some men tried to make their own hair look like a wig. Women, on the other hand, had given up their wigs of fashion—if not an artificial curl on occasion—and dressed their hair simply. Indeed, until the 1760s they kept it very close to the head—either straight or in ringlets—and covered with flounced, lace-edged caps.

Prolific experiment with the style of men's wigs makes it possible to list, at the end of the next chapter, no fewer than 110 named types. In many of these, however, the difference consists only of an extra curl here or an extra patch of frizz there. Nearly all the wigs can be considered in three main categories: full and flowing wigs, short wigs with queues and bob wigs.

Full and flowing wigs

The seventeenth-century full-bottom, most famous of the full and flowing types, lived on in the eighteenth century, remaining in favour until about 1720. It was then worn for at least a further twenty years—especially on important occasions—by old men, the aristocracy, members of professions and courtiers. Doctors were still wearing them as a matter of course in the 1730s. Were they not, as John Gay suggested, 'an index of the mind'? 'I must have a physician's habit,' says Gregory in Fielding's *The Mock Doctor*,

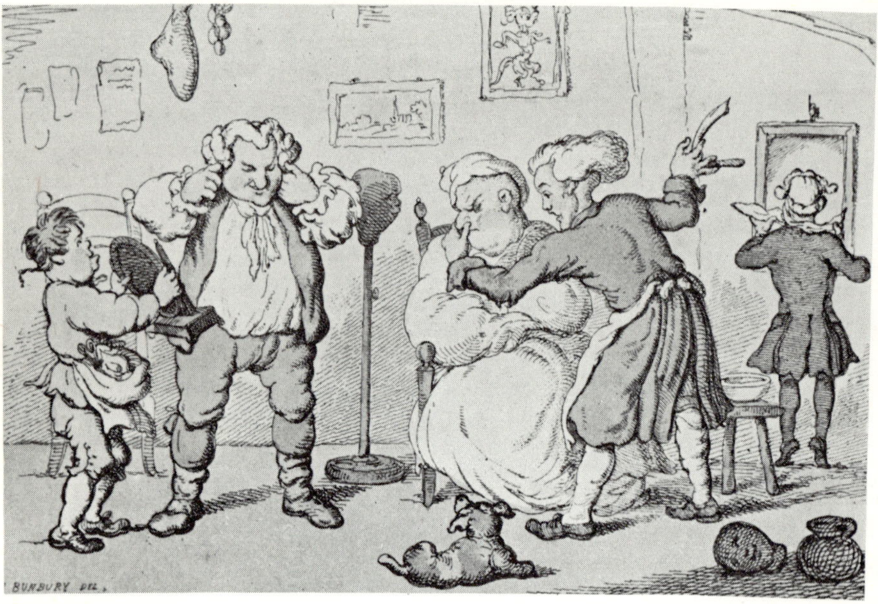

English barber's shop, *c.* 1775

1732, 'for a physician can no more prescribe without a full wig than without a fee.'

Judges never wavered in their high opinion of the full-bottom. Indeed, it is probable that they would endorse today the following line in Richard Cumberland's play of 1774, *The Choleric Man*: 'When the law lays down its full-bottomed wig, you will find less wisdom in bald pates than you are aware of.' A full-bottom is still worn by judges on the Queen's official birthday and other specially ordered days (on ordinary days they wear what is known as an undress wig, frizzed all over), and also by Queen's Counsel when pleading in the House of Lords, by the Lord Chancellor when sitting on the Woolsack and by the Speaker of the House of Commons.

The full-bottom wig reached its maximum grandeur under Queen Anne (1702–14). A fashionable kind rose in two horns above the forehead, covered the back and shoul-

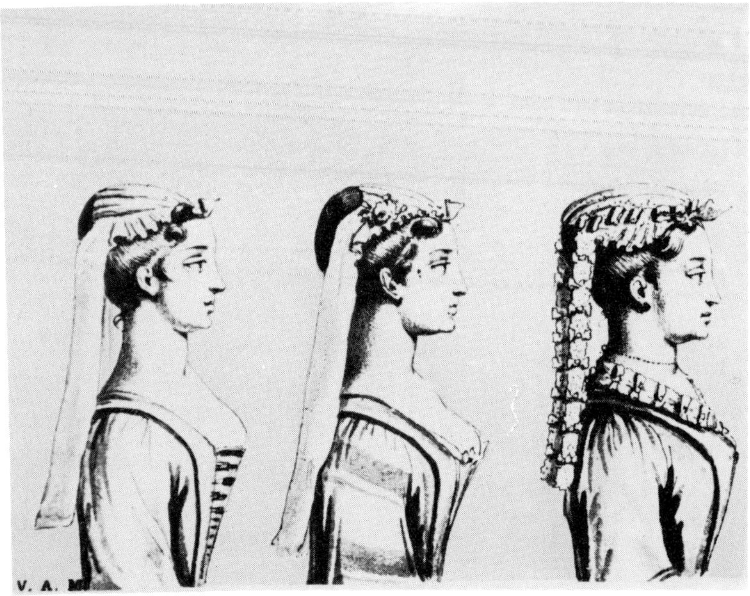

Simple hair-styles for women, 1725: drawings from the life in Bernard Lens's *The Exact Dress of the Head*

ders and flowed down upon the chest: it contained the equivalent of about ten heads of natural hair. The queen herself expressed a liking for the full-bottom and her disapproval of a growing habit among young men of wearing the small, neat tye wig. She is reported to have expressed annoyance when Eugene of Savoy, although having plenty of time to borrow the right kind of wig, insisted on appearing at an audience in a tye wig.[11]

In his *Analysis of Beauty*, William Hogarth compared the full-bottom with the lion's mane; there was something noble in it, giving 'not only dignity but sagacity to the countenance'. He also said that if it was worn much larger it would become a burlesque. Plenty of wigs in use could be said to have reached this point, though of course the broader the man the larger the wig he could carry. Tom Brown in *Letters from the Dead to the Living*, 1702, speaks of a thick-waisted man who yet 'made a most magnificent figure. His

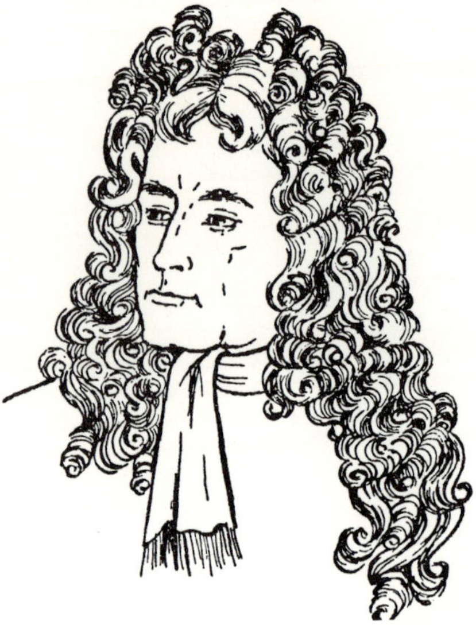

The full-bottom in the reign of Queen Anne

periwig was large enough to have loaded a camel, and he bestowed upon it at least a bushel of powder . . . he carried his hat under his left arm and walked with his hands in the waistband of his breeches.'

A type of brown full-bottom was known as the Cloudesley Shovel after Sir Cloudesley Shovel (1650–1707), Admiral of the Fleet. Its six or eight clusters of curls hanging low and brown reminded some people of loaves of bread.

The campaign wig, also called the travelling wig, was a lighter article, though certainly long and flowing. It framed the face and continued down on each side in locks eighteen inches long; but these locks, or dildos, were customarily bent up and tied. At the back a central corkscrew curl fell over the collar. The word campaign referred to the victories of Marlborough: there were also campaign coats and campaign shoes.

The adonis was a long-haired wig designed to flatter a

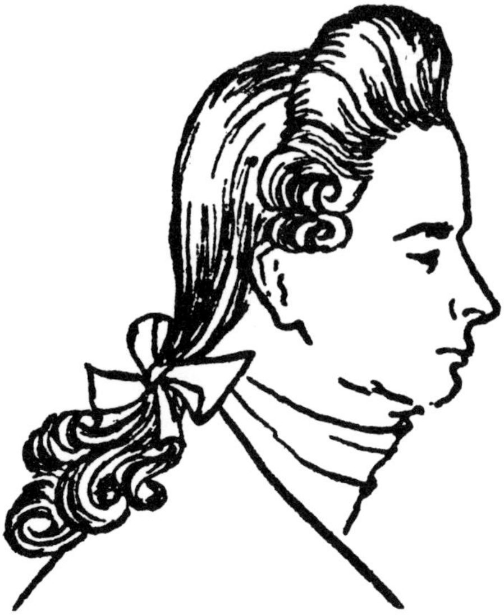

The tye wig, *c.* 1775

youthful face; it was white and had wisps that stuck out, according to the *London Magazine*, like 'the twigs of a gooseberry bush in a deep snow'.[12] In the period 1730–70 it was intermittently in favour among young men. Horace Walpole, writing to an elderly friend whose new portrait he had just seen, comments with amusement on the adonis wig he wears for it.

Short wigs with queues

These were the most stylized of the wigs and had a rather rigid appearance. A commonly-seen variety was the tye wig, in which the hair was drawn back to form a tail and then tied with black ribbon at the nape of the neck. Until about 1735 there was a suggestion of a parting in front; then it became the fashion to have a narrow roll of hair above the forehead. Sometimes a fringe of natural hair was kept so that this could be brushed and plastered up with the hair of the wig, and then given a sprinkling of powder to conceal what had happened. New arrangements for the sides of the wigs were always being introduced. Ears were normally covered. Walpole wrote in a letter of 1745 that Lord Sandwich at the Admiralty seemed to have difficulty in hearing through his wig: 'He had put on such a first-rate tye wig that nothing without the lungs of a boatswain can even think to penetrate the thickness of the curls.'

Queue wigs gradually ousted the full-bottom from the heads of merchants and men of letters. They were taken up by officers of the Navy and the Army; other ranks, when not issued with queue wigs, had to form a queue from their own hair. This was first greased and finally pipeclayed. A flash sewn to the back of the collar was intended to prevent tunics from getting stained. The wearing of queues in the services was not finally abolished until 1808.

The queue of the Ramillies wig, so named after the famous battle of 1706, was a long, gradually diminishing pigtail tied at top and tip with a bow of black ribbon. But after about 1750 the queue would be turned up and secured at the back of the neck. The queue of a wig known as temple tye or fox ear was also of pigtail length: the wig's main characteristic was a cluster of curls at the temples.

Wigs with two queues, each curled at the tip, were considered especially smart on the Continent. Denis Diderot, writing in the mid-eighteenth century, said they were to be seen everywhere in the court circles of Germany and Hungary. 'Nowadays one is unable to present oneself before the father of the Queen of Hungary without these two tails. Young and old must wear them for the great festivals and the full-dress balls.'

The major, called in France the brigadier, was a post-1750 wig with two queues tied together with a bow. It was worn by military men and by civilians affecting a military appearance. Some majors had detachable queues which enabled them, as the *London Magazine* remarked in 1764,

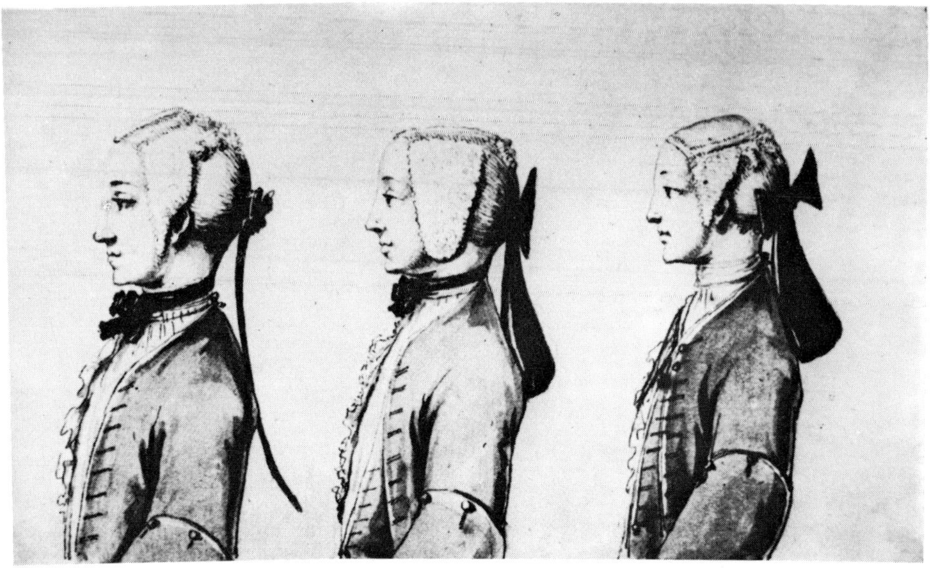

Early queue wigs, 1725. Note experiment with types of ear flap. Drawing from the life by Bernard Lens

'to do duty both at military functions and at a feast'. The Cadogan, dating from 1770, had a single generous queue which was made flat and broad, turned up on itself, and tied round the middle.

The bag wig, in use by the gentry from about 1725, had the queue enclosed in a square bag of silk or satin. The string to hold it in place was concealed by a stiff black bow at the nape of the neck. For extreme smartness, the bow could be matched by another under the chin, the two linked by a ribbon. A wig called the rose bag differed only in having its bag elaborated to look like a rose. Bags grew ever larger until they became a troublesome appendage.

Bob wigs

These were essentially short wigs without queues. They were first recorded in 1684,[13] and became popular among

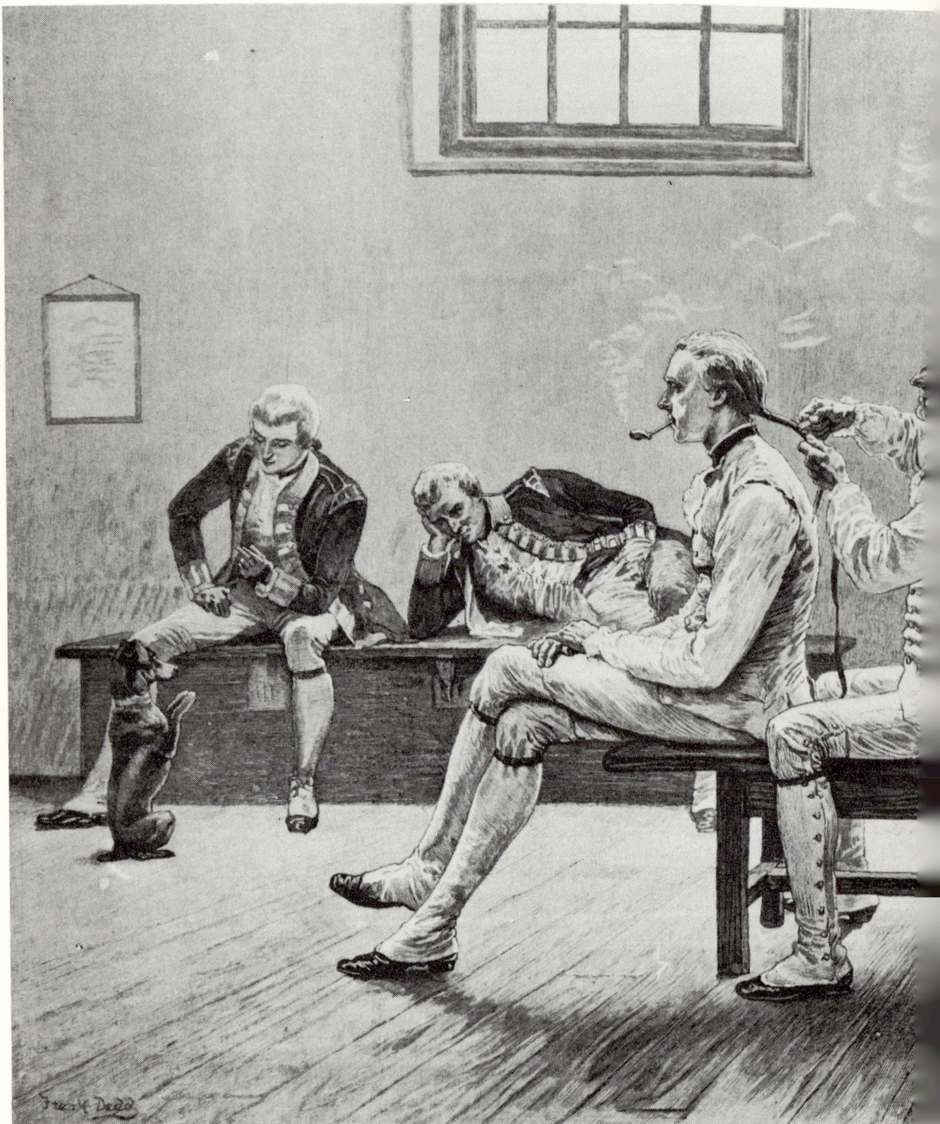

Pigtails and powder

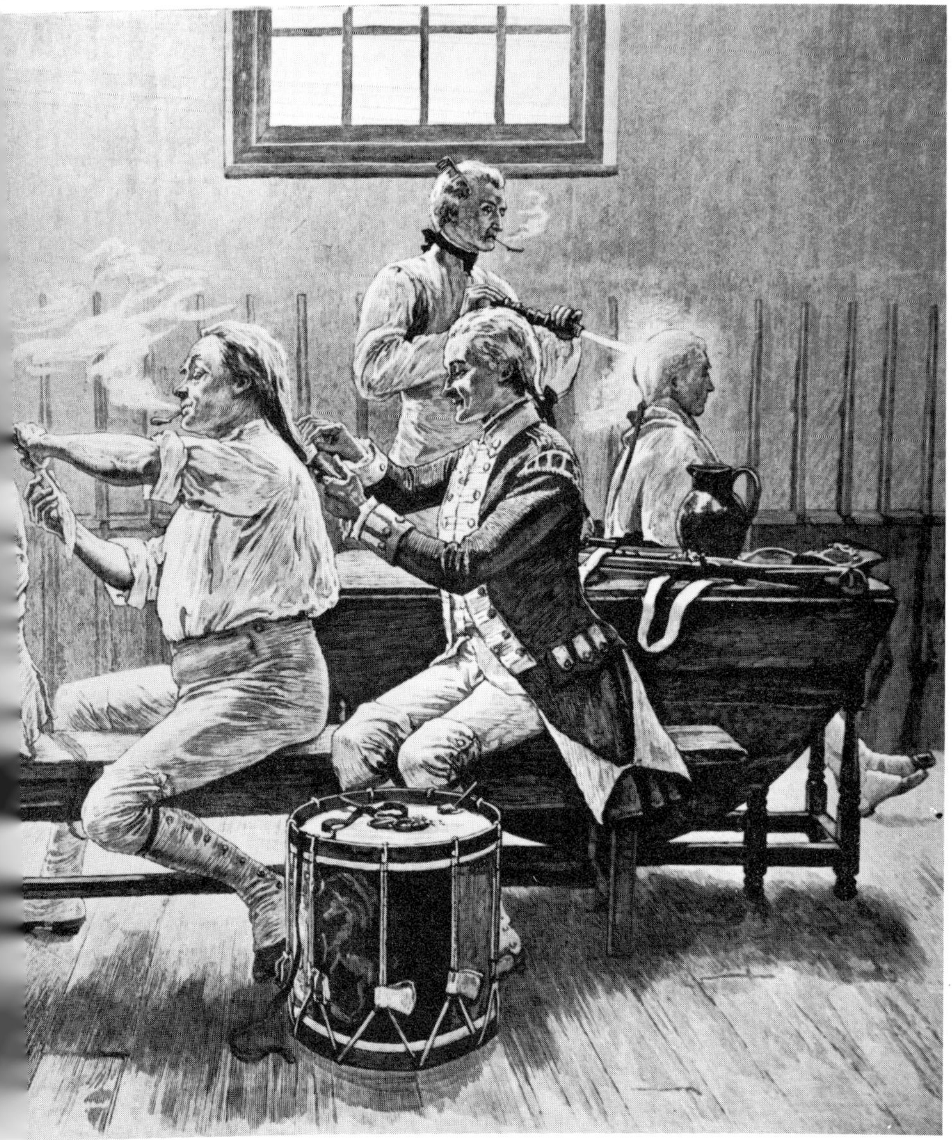

late eighteenth century

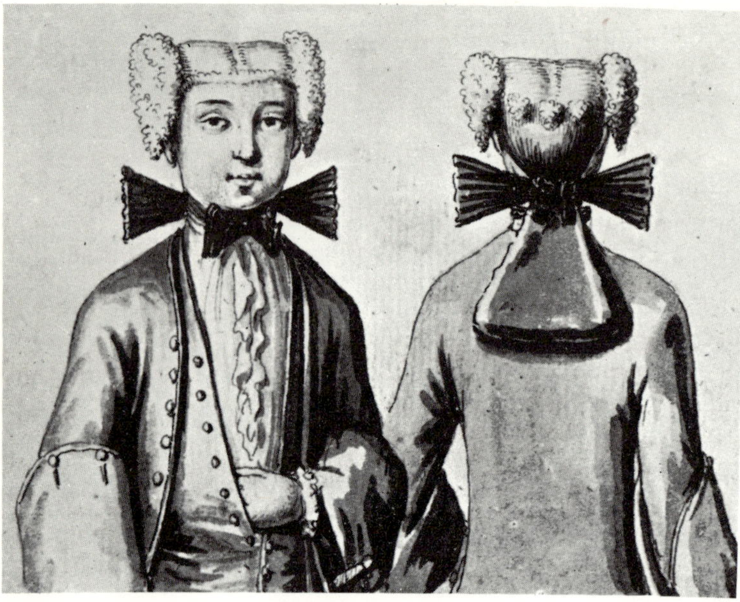

The bag wig, 1725

those who could not afford long wigs. James Stewart, a hairdresser, wrote in the 1780s of the early-eighteenth-century tradesman in his 'snug bob or natty scratch'.[14] The two main types were the long bob and the short bob, the one covering the whole of the back of the neck and the other stopping short of the nape.

Bob wigs rose steadily in the social scale. By the second half of the eighteenth century they were being made in several styles and had become good enough for anyone. An issue of the *Adventurer* in 1753 contains a description of how a 'greenhorn' becomes a 'blood': 'I cut off my hair and procured a brown bob periwig of Wilding of the same colour, with a single row of curls just round the bottom, which I wore very nicely curled and without powder.' Clergymen liked to wear bob wigs that were extra bushy, and frizzed rather than curled. A common type, the feather-top, had its crown made from the tail feathers of wild duck. Another type favoured by the clergy, and by physicians, was the aptly-named cauliflower bob. This became the usual wig for coachmen in the late eighteenth and early nineteenth century.

In the 1760s bob wigs became acceptable for full dress (they were advertised at around £1 10s). A portrait of 1768, reproduced in Mr Stevens Cox's *Dictionary of Hairdressing and Wigmaking*, shows John Harrison, horologist, wearing an elaborate bob with six rows of buckles.

Buckles, from the French *boucles*, were hollow rolls of hair which from about 1765 became a fashionable decoration for the sides of both queued and queueless wigs. Most people thought them dignified—and they were worn far into the nineteenth century. The *Gentleman's Magazine*, however, described them as 'stiff rows of curls' looking like 'gridirons', and the *London Magazine* referred to 'the immovable buckles that destroy the grace of the flowing curl'.[15]

The physical, or lion, wig was a large variety of long bob. It had the hair drawn back to a point just beyond the crown and then dressed in a puffed-out manner to the base of the neck. It was worn by physicians and other professional men, by in fact the sort of people who would formerly have worn full-bottoms. The so-called physical bush was frizzed all over. Oliver Goldsmith says of the physical wig in *The Citizen of the World*, 1762: 'To appear wise, nothing more is requisite than for a man to borrow hair from the heads of all his neighbours and clap it, like a bush, on his own; the distributors of law and physic stick on such quantities that it is almost impossible, even in idea, to distinguish between the head and the hair.'

The scratch bob was a brief and seemingly haphazard wig intended to resemble the wearer's own hair. It was much used by farmers and people with out-of-doors work. There was also, for those with the time to bother with it, a scratch wig which covered only part of the head; natural hair, should enough still grow, was swept back from the

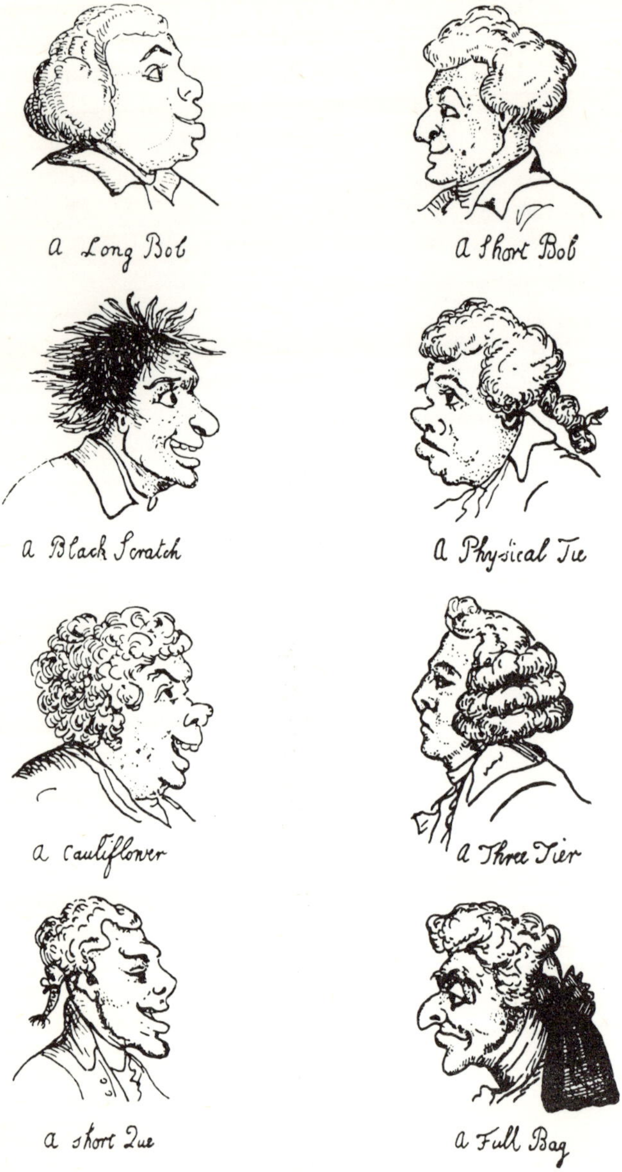

A selection of late-eighteenth-century wigs engraved by Thomas Rowlandson forehead and made to mingle with that of the wig by means of a scented grease known as pomatum. Writing in the mid-eighteenth century, John Hawkesworth remarks in *A Greenhorn to A Blood* that his hair is long enough to comb over the foretop of his scratch wig (for the evening he sometimes changed to a queue wig). There is no evidence for regarding as other than jocular a late-nineteenth-century journalist's suggestion that scratch wigs were so called because of the ease with which the hand could be slipped underneath to scratch.

One of the simplest of wigs was the cut or clipped wig. This was often worn by men servants in small households without liveried footmen. A 'Lost Servants' advertisement in the *Ipswich Journal*, 1795,[16] states: 'Servant run away in brown clipt wig, a duffel [rough wool] coat, a drill frock.' But these wigs were not confined to servants; there are several eighteenth-century references to farmers in their brown cut wigs.

Seven

Macaroni wigs, feather-tops and caxons

The Tyburn scratch, thick club and temple-tie,
The Parson's feather-top, frizzed broad and high,
The coachman's cauliflower, built tier on tiers,
Differ not more from bags and brigadiers
Than great St George's or St James's styles
From the broad dialect of broad St Giles.

G. Coleman's Prologue to *Bon Ton*, 1775

Whether smart or humble, in other words, all wigs had much in common with one another. One eighteenth-century type too fantastic to fit into the categories given was the Macaroni wig of 1773. More a male head-dress than a wig, it was dressed with a stuffing of horsehair and wool to a height of over eighteen inches. It succeeded a Macaroni fashion of 1772 for an immense knot of false hair worn at the back. Macaronis were members of the Macaroni Club, rich young men who had travelled in Italy and amused themselves with new ideas concerning dress and behaviour. Horace Walpole wrote in 1764: 'The Macaroni Club is composed of all the travelled young men who wear long curls and spying-glasses.'

The young men affected an extreme sensibility which was offended by crude tastes. They were, in fact, true dandies and fops in the eighteenth-century meaning of those words. The *Town and Country Magazine* (London) reported in 1772:[17] 'Their legs are covered with all the colours of the rainbow. Their shoes are scarce slippers and their buckles are within an inch of the toe.' Macaroni fashions spread beyond the members of the club, however, even among

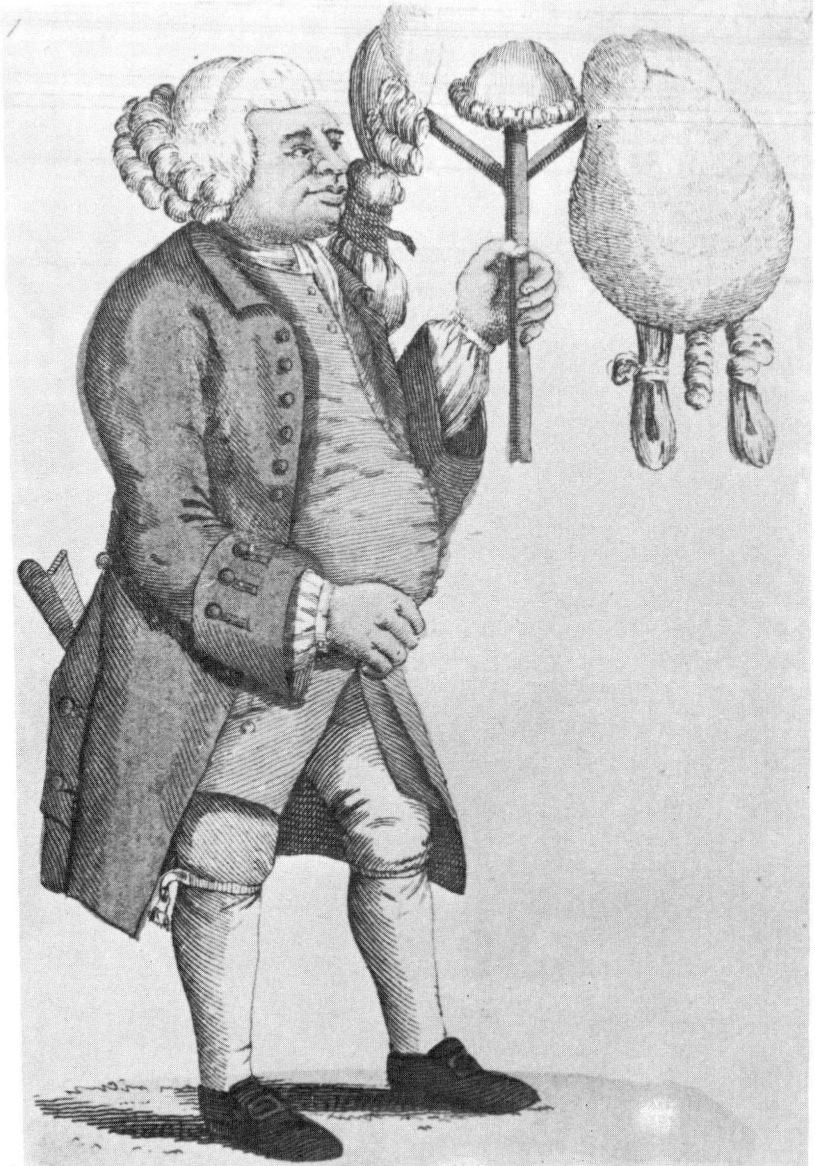

'The City Tonsor', *c.* 1770

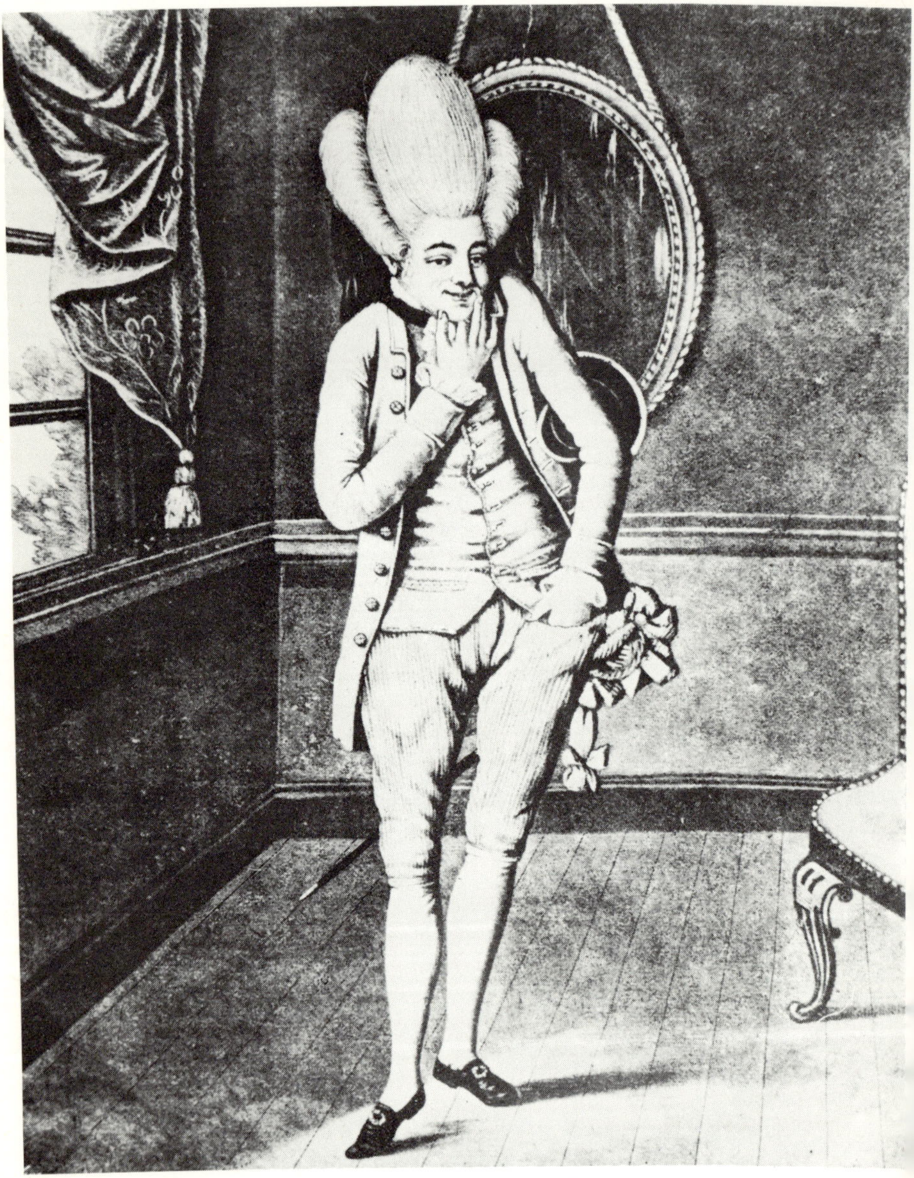

Young man with the dress and tall stuffed wig of a Macaroni, *c.* 1775

men of the Church, medicine and the law. One useful innovation was the inside breast pocket of a man's coat.

Because eighteenth-century wigs did not look like a natural growth, it has often been said that most of them were made of horsehair like the barristers' wigs of today. But all the evidence—portraits, engravings, surviving wigs—suggests that, despite the difficulty of getting enough human hair, less than half the wigs consisted of hair from horses—and from such animals as goats and cows. A list of wigs advertised in 1730 in the *London Daily Journal* specifies, at the cheaper end of the scale, 'a horse-hair tye wigg'.

There were nevertheless experimental wigs made from iron or copper wire in spiral curls. In a letter of 1751 Horace Walpole wrote as follows of Edward Wortley-Montague, son of Lady Mary Wortley: 'He diamonds himself, even to distinctive shoe buckles for a frock, and has more snuff boxes than would suffice a Chinese idol with an hundred noses. But the most curious part of his dress, which he has brought from Paris, is an iron wig; you literally would not know it from hair. I believe it is on that account that the Royal Society has just chosen him one of their body. . . .'

Feathers, sometimes used for the foretop of parsons' wigs, made also a practical material for certain sporting wigs. The *Ipswich Journal* carried an advertisement in 1750 for 'Very durable wigs, not to be hurt at least by wet, made of the single feathers in mallards' tails'. The same paper refers in 1761 to 'Gentlemen's perukes for sporting made of drakes' tails'.[18]

Cork wigs were so called because of their lightness, according to Mr Stevens Cox, not because cork came into their construction. Mr Stevens Cox quotes a reference of 1785 to 'the cork bob, that sits so snug and tight, whose light formation wraps a head as light. . . .' He also quotes this announcement in the *Salisbury Journal*, 1763: 'John Light, peruke maker, has brought to great perfection the best method of making cork wigs, either smooth or in curls and also cork bag-wigs in the neatest manner.'

When a wig had no style, any recognizable design having disappeared through neglect or the effects of bad weather, it would be referred to, even by its owner, as a caxon; the name—originally caxton—came into being when a murderer who disguised himself in a wig was hanged and exposed on the gibbet near the town of Caxton in Cambridgeshire.

William Woty[19] devoted nearly two pages in *The Shrubs of Parnassus*, 1760, to the rugged charm of the caxon. He maintained that with a 'snowwhite shirt' and a shilling in his pocket he could go out in his caxon and feel quite at ease among beaux in silken bag wigs and barristers in consequential tyes. 'I too can strut, and sip my coffee down, And mingle in the Mall without a blush.' It amuses him to dwell at length on the damage done to fashionable wigs by wind, rain and snow—and by failing to support them carefully overnight. Need I tell you, asks Woty, how different it is with a caxon,

> How, when I regulate its rumpled form,
> I dash it on a post with stroke oblique,
> Or full direct upon a table's verge?
> Need I recite the dangers it has passed,
> How yet it reigns secure?

At the end of the eighteenth century, when wigs were going out of fashion, the term caxon came to be a colloquialism for any wig, rather as any tall bicycle was dubbed a penny-farthing when this type was becoming old-fashioned. 'Caxon' was even used quite seriously for types of cauliflower and tye wig worn by coachmen and certain professional men.

There follows a list, taken from Mr Stevens Cox's *Dictionary of Hairdressing and Wigmaking*, of the named wigs thrown up by the seventeenth and eighteenth centuries. Wig names from France, such as *perruque à la cavalière*

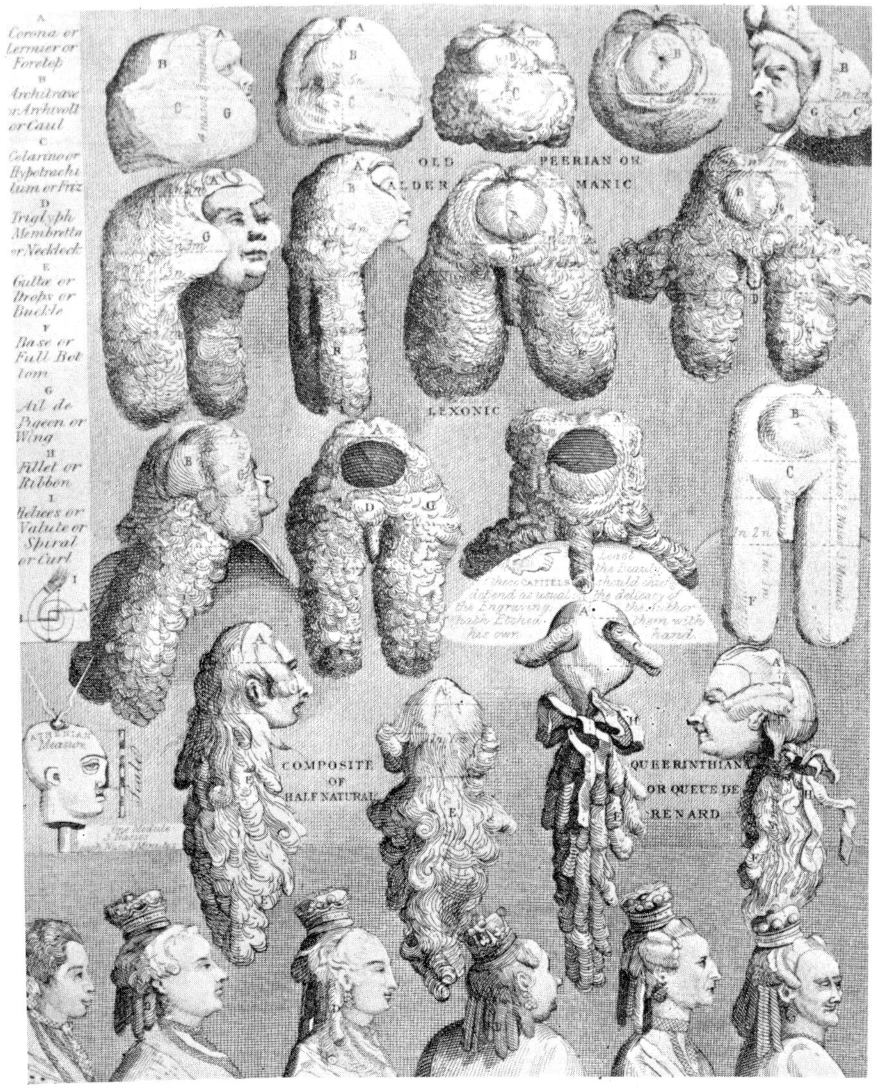

William Hogarth's 'The five Orders of Perriwigs as they were worn at the late Coronation [that of George III] measured architectonically'

and *perruque à l'aventure* have been shortened to cavalière and aventure. Unexpected contemporary spellings have been kept.

Men's—seventeenth century

Allonge
Barrister's
Brown George or
Cloudesley Shovel
Cadanette
Duvillier or furbelow
Full-bottom
Gregorian
Military
Puff

Men's—eighteenth century

Adonis
Adorable
Albemarle
Aldermanic
Allegrec
Anvieu
Apothecary's grizzled
Aventure
Bag
Bishop's
Black riding
Bob
Bob major
Bonnet
Brigadier
Brush
Brutus
Busby
Bush
Buzz
Cabriolet
Cadogan or club
Campaign
Cap
Cauliflower
Chain buckle
Chancellor
Chasseur
Chizzled
Club
Cork
Curled bob
Dalmahoy
Detached buckle
Double queued
Dragonne
Drop lock
Ecconomme
Elephant
Entiquitee
Dutch
Fantail
Favorie
Feather top
Felicite
Fox ear
Francoise
Frizz
Full bob
Full dress bob
Gendarme
Gentilly
Grecian fly
Gregorian
Hedgehog
Impassiant
Inconstance
Indifference
Italienne
Jalousie
Legere
Lion
Long bob
Long queue
Louis
Lunatique
Macaroni
Maitre d'hotel
Maw-worm
Naissante
Natural

Natural fly
Naud espagnol
Negligent
Nouvelle mode
Ordinaire
Oyseau Royale
Paresseuse
Parisienne
Pattes de lapin
Pendant bob
Petit maitre
Physical
Physical tye
Pigeon's wing
Pigtail
Port Mahou
Prudence Puff
Ramillies
Ravir
Relisle
Rhinoceros
Rose bag
Royale
Savage black
Scratch
Scratch bob
She-dragon
Short queue
Singuliere
Spencer
Squared
Staircase
Temple-tye
Tronchin
Tuck
Twist
Tyburn scratch
Tye
Vallancy
Vieillard

Women's—eighteenth century

Belle Poule
Caracalla
Charmes de la Liberté
Diadem
Medusa
Minerve
Marchioness
Royal Bird

Eight

Life with a wig

Eighteenth-century wigs were worn with so casual a panache they could be lifted in public to scratch the shaved head. Alderman Boydell, a respected publisher who became Lord Mayor of London, used to hang his wig daily on top of a pump in Ironmonger Lane while he washed his head beneath the spout.[20] London had countless pumps.

Removal of the wig on formal occasions was unusual (Horace Walpole removed his wig more than once in the House of Commons), but it did come off, if the room was not too draughty, for sitting at ease with old friends.* Some houses had wall pegs for visitors' wigs in the entrance hall. Wigs were taken off as a matter of course before a 'bout of fisticuffs': hence the expression 'keep your wig on' for 'don't get excited'. And a man doing exacting or strenuous manual work—a surgeon, say, or a blacksmith—normally did it bareheaded. In *Humphry Clinker*, 1771, Smollett narrates that a surgeon 'laying aside his cap and periwig, equipped himself with a night cap, apron and sleeves'.

It could be different for people working in the open air in cold weather. Pehr Kalm, a Swede who went to England in 1748, saw labourers in wigs working in the fields. He noted in his book *Visit to England* that wigs were worn by 'farm servants, clodhoppers, day labourers—all labouring people'. As the cheapest wig cost at least a guinea,† and farm workers'

* The London *Hairdressers' Weekly Journal* in an article of 1886 said that men who had gone bald would sometimes guard against embarrassing accidents by wearing an inner wig simulating stubble. No evidence is to be found for the assertion

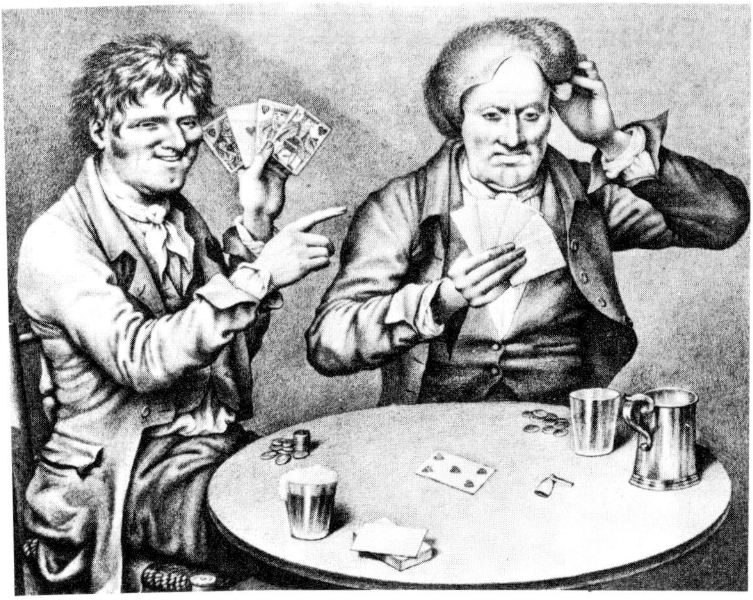

Wigs could be lifted to scratch the head

wages were about eight shillings a week, it is likely that Kalm was in fact writing only of men on particular estates where the wigs for the squire and his household were so often changed that used ones were distributed among the outside workers. In Farquhar's *The Beaux' Strategem*, 1707, a servant is mistaken for a captain on account of his 'fine long periwig tied up in a bag'.

Having laid aside their wigs—for one reason or another—most men liked to cover the head with a night cap. A cap of fine material was worn as a matter of course by the man of rank at the times when he considered he was not dressed. He might spend the first few hours of the day in a state of 'undress'—that is, in casual clothes and with his face and

† Thomas Turner, a retired grocer living quietly in Sussex, mentioned in his diary in 1746 that he paid £1 15s for 'a new wigg'—Ralph Edwards, *English Furniture*, Country Life, 1964

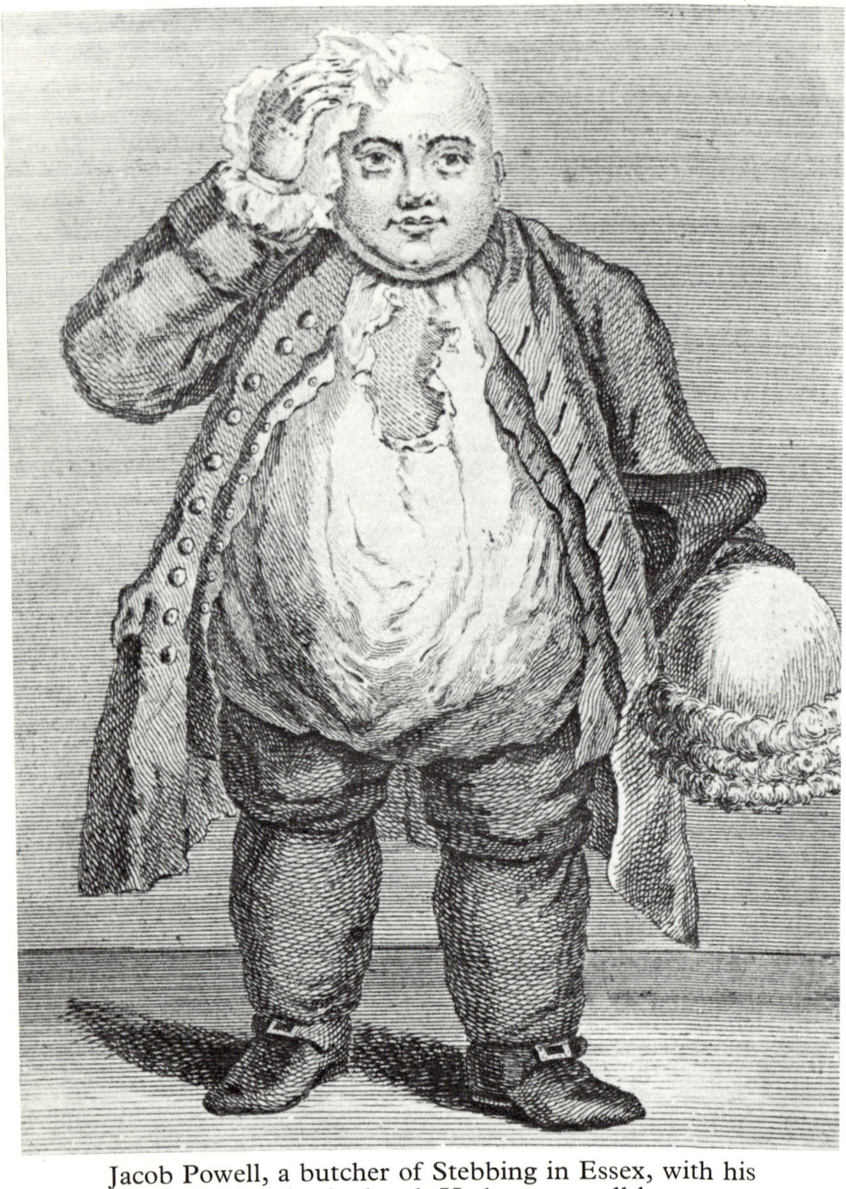

Jacob Powell, a butcher of Stebbing in Essex, with his three-tier bob in the hand. He became well known on account of his size—he died in 1754 aged 37 and weighing just under 40 stone head unadorned. Then he would have his servant help him set about the ritual of preparing him from top to toe for the eyes of the world. It was a ritual which could last two hours, even a whole morning in the opinion of a writer for the London *Connoisseur* of October 1754: 'The gentlemen too will have their toilettes set out with washes, perfumes, and cosmetics; and will spend a whole morning in scenting their linen, dressing their hair, and arching their eyebrows.'

Night caps for undress use were often called morning caps. There were two styles, one with a tall crown and a flat turned-down brim, the other with a shapeless crown and a rolled brim; the latter flopped to one side and would be decorated with a tassel. There were also wigs, cap-like in form, which were used with undress, especially a type of simple bob wig. Well known men often sat for their portraits in undress, with a night cap instead of a wig on their heads. Even the statue of Sir John Powell, a judge who died in 1713, shows him, not in his habitual long-bottom wig, but in a skull cap.[21] The reason is well explained in the *Spectator* of 28 July 1712:

> Great masters in painting never care for drawing people in the fashion; as very well knowing that the head-dress or periwig that now prevails and gives a grace to their portraitures at present, will make a very odd figure and perhaps look monstrous in the eyes of posterity. For this reason they very often represent an illustrious person in a Roman habit, or in some other dress that never varies.[22]

A similar wish for portraiture not to become dated influenced Roman sculptors; some of the busts had the hair worked in a different coloured marble which could be removed. The bust of Plautilla in the Louvre has a detachable marble wig.

On the Continent wig-wearing was confined more to men of education, and among these in certain countries it was *de rigueur*. Friedrich Nicolai, in his history of wigs published

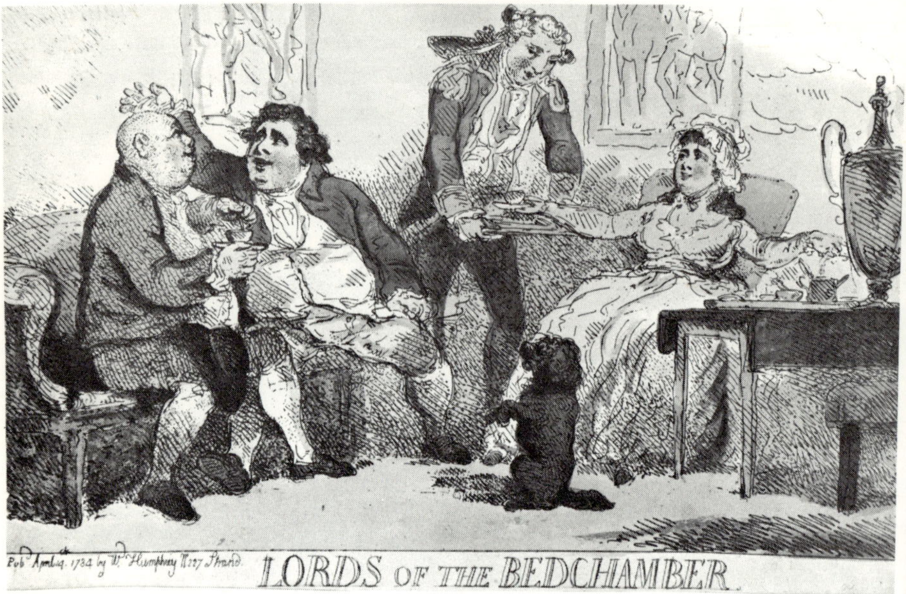

The Duchess of Devonshire sees a visitor's wig playfully knocked off by Charles James Fox. Print of 1784

in 1801,[23] said it was rare by the middle of the eighteenth century to see a single student at Halle, or any other German university, who was wearing his own hair.

In several of the German dukedoms wigs were made to carry a tax. Wig-wearing Berliners were taxed from as early as 1698. But a wig tax instituted in Prussia in 1704 was abolished in 1717 by King Frederick William I. This was not, however, to encourage the wearing of wigs: on the contrary, the king deplored the large sums of money spent on what he considered a stupid extravagance.

On his first day as king, according to Nicolai's account, Frederick William discharged eighty-eight heavily bewigged chamberlains. And within a few months he himself ceased to wear a wig. He wore military uniform all the time, combing his hair flat and drawing it into a small queue at the back. Louis XV of France liked at about this time (1720–5) to tear off people's wigs, according to Barbier's

53

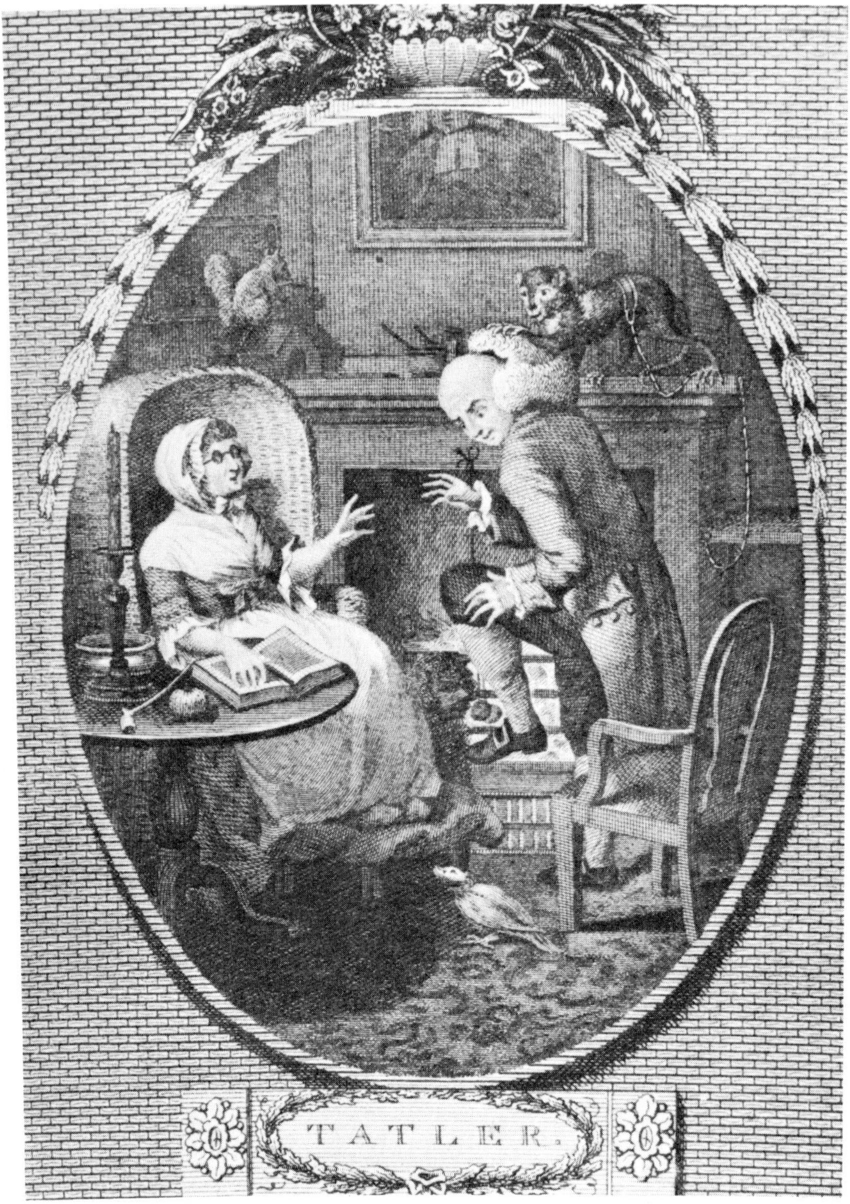

Long bob interfered with by monkey, *c.* 1785

Journal,[24] but this was the malicious trick of an indulged young man (it also amused him to snatch away people's canes) and not an action inspired by any dislike of wigs. Except for Frederick William, all the kings and princes of Europe wore wigs, and so did the officers of all armies other than those serving Frederick William.

In Paris even children had wigs. The historian Mercier considered this was going too far and commented that monkeys dancing on cords were not more ridiculous. He described the carefully nurtured Parisian boy of seven, wigged and powdered. He would wear a full-sleeved and broad-skirted coat, immense ruffles and a needle of a sword on his thigh, and with a cocked hat under his arm he would hold himself erect and bow like a judge. He seemed to have neither wrists, arms nor legs of his own, but he had been taught how to sit down and how to walk a minuet. If he ever met English boys, he made an irresistible target for their mockery.

In England a smart lady might buy a periwig for her page, or a man for his little son—especially if the child was to have a portrait sitting*—but in general wigs were not for children. It was a matter for comment, though, if a young man over seventeen was still wearing his own hair.

Men wore wigs of natural colours until about 1714 when it became fashionable to bleach them; but a bleached wig soon faded and ceased to look fresh. It became the custom to coat the hair with a scented powder: this might consist of finely ground starch or flour or of mineral substances—even gold dust. Putting powder on hair was not new. It is reported that some of Louis XIV's younger courtiers, copying actors, used to dust their heads with sweet-smelling starch. Louis disliked the habit for aesthetic reasons, only in old age permitting a light sprinkling of white on his black wig; Louis XV wore powder on his head from childhood.[25]

The powdering operation, ideally a job for an attendant,

* Lord Bristol spent £2 3s in 1698 on a wig for a son aged 11—according to a record quoted by Ralph Edwards, op. cit.

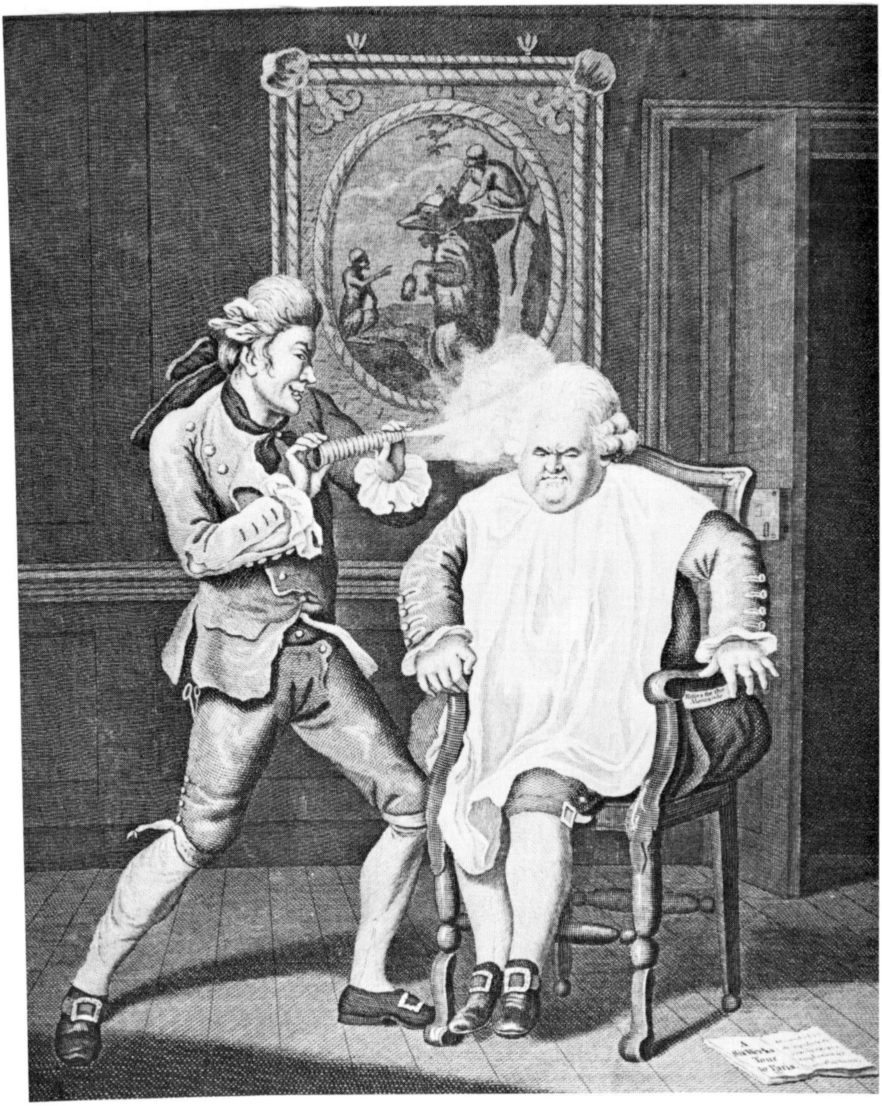

'The Englishman in Paris', 1770

was carried out either with a bellows or a large powder puff. The man being powdered would wear a powdering jacket and, if he was wise, protect his face and eyes with a paper mask or a funnel-shaped paper nosebag. Big houses might have a room set aside for the work known as a wig closet. Parson Woodforde, who did his own powdering, recorded in 1789: 'For a powder puff for my Wiggs pd 2s.'

As the century advanced, powder was applied ever more lavishly, the hair having been liberally greased to encourage it to stick. Grey and white were the colours mainly used at first and were those which remained popular; but brown was not unusual and blue, violet, pink and yellow powders were tried. Plenty of men liked the light powders because they flattered the face and made the eyes brighter; it was the men—before the women—who discovered that a lavish application of grey or white powder eliminated one of the signs of age, grey or white hair. Even young men made their wigs as light as possible for the sake of the becoming effect. This could be annoying to older people. The Reverend John Tomlinson wrote in his *Diary* in 1718: 'Uncle found fault with my wig for being so light.'[26]

Wig-wearing was so much a part of everyday life that a move to leave them off in the 1760s represented a big change in manners. Mostly it was young men who rebelled, but the old, too—especially those who had perfectly good hair of their own beneath their wigs—tried the experiment of going without a wig. A social effect is illustrated in this passage from Parson Woodforde's *Diary* for 1764: 'Old Mr Dalton and his son called on me this morning . . . I did not know old Mr Dalton at first, as he now wears his hair.' A professor of divinity at Oxford, Dr Randolph, even appeared in his own hair when he kissed hands with the monarch on being appointed to a bishopric. 'You have got no wig!' exclaimed George III. 'Don't you mean to have a wig?' Dr Randolph's answer in the negative was swept aside. 'You *must* have a wig,' said the king.[27]

Many whose own hair was sparse, a not unusual condition after years of wig-wearing, felt obliged to conceal the fact. In John Macdonald's *Memoirs of an Eighteenth Century Footman*[28] there is an account of James Coutts, the banker, having tried twenty servants in one month before finding a man who could dress him to his liking. He wore what is now called a hair-piece to supplement his own hair. 'It required', said Macdonald (who got the job), 'a person that understood the business of wig-making. When he was dressed no person could tell there was anything but his own hair. . . .'

The move away from wigs greatly upset the great band of wigmakers; many of them, with no work to do, were going through acute hardship. In February of 1765 the wigmakers of London actually petitioned George III, drawing his attention to distress following 'the decline of the trade occasioned by the present mode of men in all stations wearing their own hair', and begging him to bring back the wig. If the wigmakers' petition had nothing to do with male wigs largely coming back at the end of the 1760s, their movement in procession to St James's caused a memorable stir.

As the wigmakers marched along, it was noticed, according to both Horace Walpole and Press accounts of the day, that most of them were not themselves wearing wigs; and the sight so affected sections of the watching mob that all wigless barbers were seized and forcibly denuded of their natural hair.

Wigs began finally to go out of fashion in the 1790s. The change was hastened by serious rebellion in France (where the wig was seen as a badge of the aristocracy) and by the English government's decision in 1795 to levy a tax of a guinea a year on hair-powdering. In the initial year this yielded £20,000, a considerable sum at the time. In Hull, it was stated in the local newspaper, over 900 hair-powder certificates were issued in the first two months of the tax becoming effective. But receipts soon began to fall. The Duke of Bedford, protesting about this levy by Pitt's government, was one of the first to put aside his wig and start wearing his hair cropped and unpowdered. In the

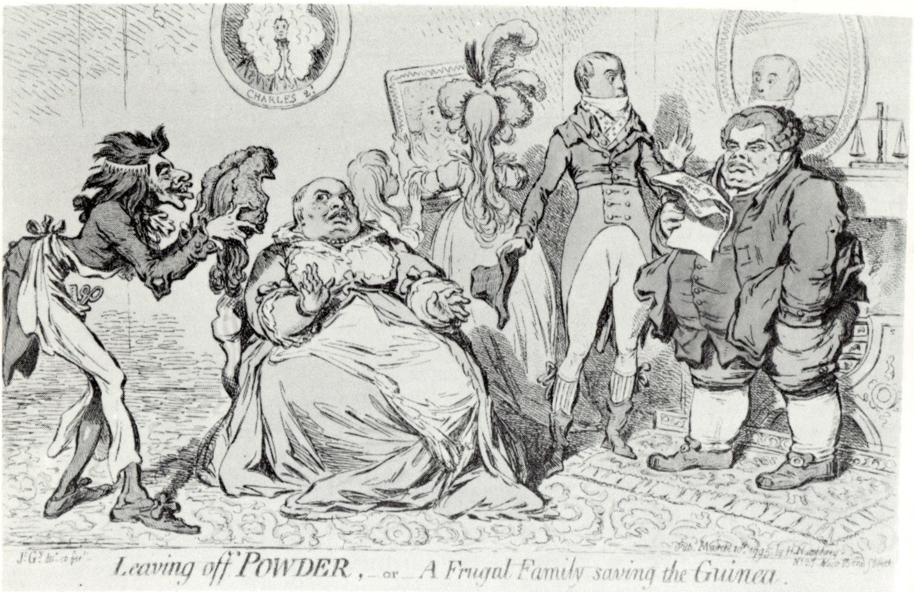

It was a shock at first to see the natural colour of hair. But those who paid the powder tax of 1795 were known as guinea pigs

spring of 1795, *The Times* was able to report:

> A club has been formed called the Crop Club, every member of which is obliged to have his head cropped for the purpose of evading the tax on powdered heads . . . the new crop is called the Bedford level.

One of the last of the wigs to be launched was the Brutus, which was brown and untidy: it was derived from the Brutus haircut affected in France at a time when the ideal was Empire and the victorious Roman.

By the year 1801 it was correct for gentlemen to wear their hair very short, a mode which those who lived in great houses would not permit, however, for their footmen. For these the wig lingered on until well into the nineteenth century and was replaced by powdered hair which lasted, for the smartest footmen, until around 1900. In the 1880s a silk bow would be fixed at the back of the neck of the coat to represent the bow of a non-existent wig.[29] But as late as 1886, according to an article of that year in the *Hairdressers' Weekly Journal*, there were still a few coachmen and servants in livery who wore wigs.

Otherwise—at the beginning of the nineteenth century—only clergymen, doctors and lawyers remained faithful to a fashion which had been almost universal throughout Europe and America for nearly a century and a half.

Nine

The early fashion wigs of America

Wigs had arrived in America by the end of the 1660s. They were introduced by officials of the king and soon taken up by the more well-to-do of the settlers; what was the correct mode in England had also to be the mode in the wilderness.

Many a Puritan preacher denounced wig-wearing from the pulpit, declaring it had 'no warrant in the word of God'. John Eliot, the Massachusetts missionary to the Indians, maintained that the calamities suffered by the colonists in their war with the Indians, known as King Philip's War, were a divine punishment for wearing false hair. Increase Mather, the celebrated Puritan minister, raged against wigs in Boston, where they were particularly fashionable. His own son, Cotton Mather, wore one. So did a large number of students at Harvard, and also (from the year 1670) the governor of New Hampshire.

None of the abuse to which wearers of wigs were subjected checked the fashion. In the southern colonies wigs came to be worn almost as generally as in England—by blacksmiths, innkeepers and bricklayers as well as by rich Virginian planters and clergymen. To start with wigs were ordered from London, but local barbers set about making themselves familiar with wigmaking. Such was the demand for wigs that numbers of London wigmakers emigrated with a view to practising their craft more profitably in the American colonies. Here is a typical advertisement in a New York paper of 1761:

> Morrison, peruke maker from London, dresses ladies and gentlemen's hair in the politest taste. He has a choice parcel of human, horse and goat's hair to dispose of.

It was customary for common barbers, until at least 1800, to include tooth-drawing among their services, but the following New York announcement of 1768 was unusual:

> James Daniel, wigmaker and hairdresser also operates on the teeth, a business so necessary in this city.

In 1769 the small town of Williamsburg, capital of Virginia, had eight wigmakers. The colony of New York levied a tax on wigs without any noticeable check on the flow of orders for new wigs or for renovating worn ones. Wigmakers would often be hired by the month or the year to keep their handiwork in good condition and gladly undertook a house-to-house service.

'On a Saturday afternoon,' writes Leonard E. Fisher, historian of the American wigmakers, 'it was not unusual to see scores of wigmakers' apprentices dashing through the narrow streets of Boston, or any other early American city, rushing to deliver the freshly curled and powdered wigs belonging to the great and near-great men of the day. The careful workmanship of the wigmaker was demanded of

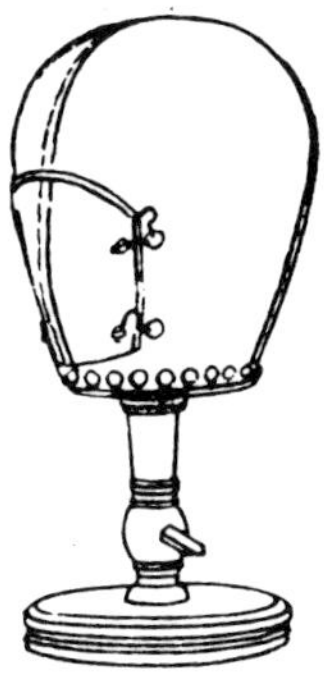

Mid-eighteenth-century leather wig block on wooden stand—in the collection of Edward Pinto and one of the illustrations in John Gloag's *Short Dictionary of Furniture*, Allen & Unwin, 1969 edition. Note small door allowing wigmaker to keep tools within the head

him by colonial people who took pride in their appearance. It was the pride of those who valued their place in the life of a new and promising nation.'[30]

The era of men's wigs as part of dress came to an end in America at about the same time as in England. The wig-making business declined steadily after the War of Independence had been won in 1783. As in France, a new way of life was beginning.

On both sides of the Atlantic wig-wearing made a mark on the history of furniture; for just as farthingales and hooped skirts brought into being certain types of chair, so wigs caused cabinet makers to produce wig blocks, wig boxes and wig stands which are still to be seen.

A wig block is a head represented in wood or leather—or both—with a brief, circular-based stand; on it a wig would be made and subsequently dressed and repaired. A wig box is a container of wood or pasteboard with a carrying handle which is fitted with a support in the shape of a mushroom. A wig stand, or table, denotes a small turned baluster finishing in a bulbous knob—considerably smaller than a

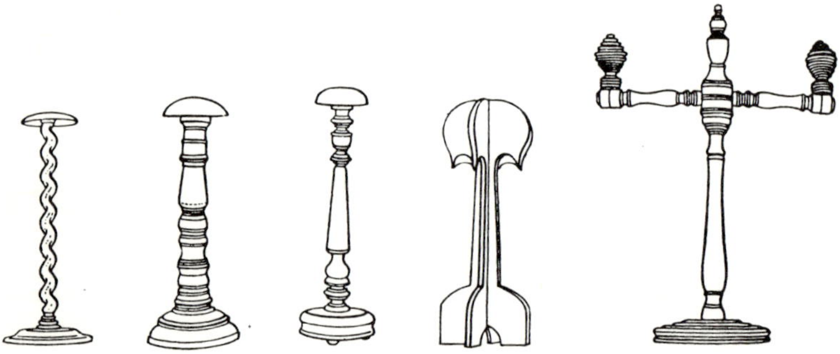

Wig stands in wood in the collection of Edward Pinto and illustrating John Gloag's *Short History of Furniture*, Allen & Unwin, 1969 edition. First article, twist-turned: 1660–70. Second and third: mid-eighteenth century. Fourth, a travelling model which could be dismantled for packing flat: late eighteenth century. Fifth, a double stand: late eighteenth or early nineteenth century wig block—on which a wig could be hung. The base is usually circular. Some of these stands consisted of four wings, fitted together, enabling the stand to be taken apart and packed flat for travelling. Others had two arms fitted with turned cones to take two wigs. Most surviving wig stands belong to the late eighteenth century: the turning of the balusters, which may look earlier, cannot be relied on as a guide to date, for traditional forms were used.

The terms 'wig stand' and 'wig table' are often applied wrongly to a light tripod stand of mahogany made to hold a basin and fitted with small drawers:[31] it was designed simply as a wash-basin stand. The water jug stood on a hollow platform below the top. The association with wigs seems to have arisen through the stand having sometimes been used to hold powder and utensils connected with their use.

Ten

Making a head

Peruke Maker, makes all sorts of false hair for ladies' tetes, tupees, braids, curls.

Salisbury Journal, 1771

The wigmakers need not have worried about the men's fashion of the mid-1760s to do without a wig. As it turned out, women were on the point of adopting a French mode of arranging the hair which was to bring them unprecedented wealth—not so much through a demand for complete wigs as for quantities of false hair to be mixed with the natural. Women's hair, after a century of being dressed close to the scalp, was now beginning to rise.

At first only the hair in front rose, dressed over pads. Then, in the second half of the 1760s, came the têtes: the whole head of hair was widened and built up in a tower to a height of twelve inches above the scalp. In the 1770s it was known to reach to a height of two feet six inches—a phenomenon noted in numerous contemporary cartoons. The Empress Maria Theresa wrote in 1775 to her daughter Marie Antoinette, wife of Louis XVI: 'They say that your coiffure rises thirty six inches . . . and is decorated with a mass of feathers and ribbons, which make it even higher . . . I was always of the opinion that one should follow the fashions with restraint but never exaggerate them.'[32] But Marie Antoinette had as hairdresser le Grand Leonard, and if part of her tête had to be lifted off every time she wished to enter her carriage, that was a small payment for being an accepted leader of fashion. At least some of the

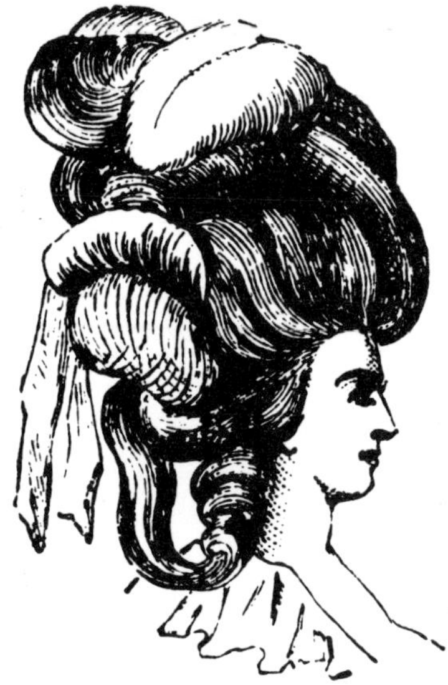

Great quantities of false hair were mixed with the natural

door openings at Versailles were raised to accommodate tall heads.

To achieve the fashionable tête there had to be an elaborate framework of padding consisting of greased wool with horsehair. The natural hair was built up on this as far as it would go, plastered down with paste or pomatum, and then supplemented by several times its amount by false hair. A rich woman could well spend half a day with her hairdresser, 'making a head'. Even those unable to command the attentions of a hairdresser struggled nevertheless to adopt 'Frenched' hair. A newspaper advertisement of 1778 drew attention to a 'new invented Elastic Cushion' which was said to be 'very convenient for ladies that dress their own hair, as they require but few or no pins'. But pins, single or double, normally had to be used; they were very long pins and sometimes set with diamonds, pearls or garnets.

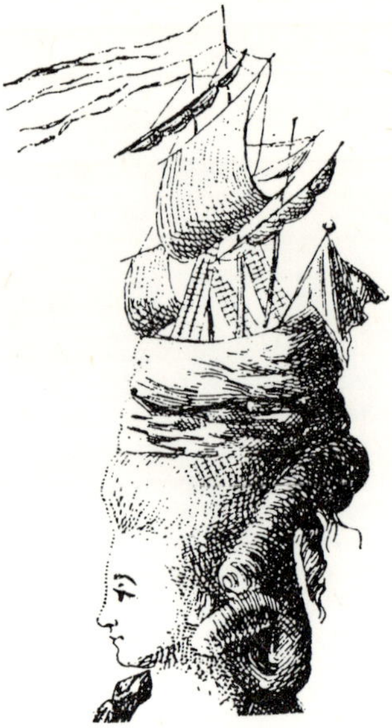

Coiffure à la Belle Poule

Ornaments for the lofty heads of hair included vegetables, fruits, feathers and baskets of flowers. Sometimes the flowers were provided with water. 'I wore in my hair', writes Mme d'Oberkirch in her *Memoirs*, 'little flat bottles shaped to the curvature of the head; into these a little water was poured for the purpose of preserving the freshness of the natural flowers . . . This did not always succeed, but when it did, the effect was charming. Nothing could be more lovely than the floral wreath crowning the snowy pyramid of powdered hair.'

In France, some of the hair ornaments were inspired by political events. In 1778, for instance, following a flashy sea battle in which the ship *La Belle Poule* engaged the English, women took to crowning their hair with a model of a frigate in full sail and complete with cannons and flags. The models were by no means pocket-sized.

Even without the need to keep the head upright in order

not to upset the flower water, the bother and inconvenience of wearing tall hair was considerable. A correspondent of the *Lady's Magazine* had this to say in March 1776:[33]

> I have seen several ladies, very handsome, so disguised and features quite distorted, by the horrid drag of their hair to a height absolutely half as tall as themselves, and so loaded with game, flowers, fruit, herbs, ribbons, pins, etc . . . that it has really seemed a pain for them to move or speak for fear the wonderful building be demolished.

Moving and speaking were easy, given reasonable headroom, compared with going to bed, passing through doorways (it was not only at Versailles that some of these were raised) and riding in carriages. The caricaturists of the period had no need to call on their imaginations to depict women in ridiculous postures. Looking about them in the streets they could see, as everyone else could see, that the lady of quality going by in her sedan chair was not sitting in it, she was squatting on the floor.

The *Gentleman's and London Magazine*[34] reported in 1777 that the seats of coaches were sunk almost to the bottom, and that though women sat with their knees up to the pits of their stomachs, they were still obliged to bend forwards to avoid touching the roof. 'Yet they are not to be talked out of this absurdity. The fashion is likely to last.'

It lasted for a good ten years more. Even Nancy Woodforde, a vicar's niece living in a remote Norfolk vicarage, was dressing her hair in the tall French manner in 1782—according to Parson Woodforde's reference in his *Diary* to her acquisition of a cushion on which to arrange it.

Catching fire was more than a remote possibility in times when reception rooms were lighted with chandeliers holding dozens of candles. The point is brought out by

Christopher Anstey in his *New Bath Guide* of 1776:

> Yet Miss at the rooms
> Must beware of her plumes;
> For if Vulcan her feather embraces,
> Like poor Lady Laycock
> She'll burn like a haycock,
> And roast all the Loves and the Graces.

A degree of discomfort was taken for granted, however. Anna Green Winslow,[35] in a diary entry for 1771, referred to the effect of building up her hair on a roll consisting of cow's tail and coarse horsehair: 'It makes my head ache and burn and itch like anything.'

Having once made a smart head, women were naturally reluctant to take it down. By sleeping in a specially propped-up position, it could be made to last a week; though by that time dismantlement was a matter of urgency. Combing to give elementary hygiene was not possible, and washing the hair was still a twice-yearly event. In a letter of 1767, the Countess of Suffolk records hearing someone remark to Lord Chesterfield that women at Bath seemed to be wearing their hair 'three or four storeys high'. Lord Chesterfield replied: 'Yes, and I believe every storey is inhabited, like the lodging houses here, for I observe a great deal of scratching.'[36]

The ivory or silver scratching stick of the period, with its end in the form of a human hand, was for scratching backs rather than heads; for the latter a simple pin of some kind was more practical. Scratching of course was a feeble palliative. Many women had their heads shaved and wore complete wigs in the hairstyle of the day; however, this was not considered entirely *comme il faut* and such wigs were worn with secrecy.

Around 1780 women's hair decreased in height but increased in width. The back part was done in a chignon and hung in a flat loop from the top of the head to the shoulders; otherwise it might be plaited. The towering head-dress persisted longer in France than in England. Madame Dubarry wore it, as did everyone at Court, throughout the decade prior to the Fall of the Bastille in 1789. Ornamentation of the head was consistently eye-catching.

To understand why English women gave themselves to so ridiculous a fashion it is only necessary to remember the strength of French influence and to read of the extreme seriousness with which anything to do with hairdressing was taken in France. From early in the eighteenth century the more dexterous women's hairdressers were idolized; they were the spoiled children of the ladies of the Court and of the rich bourgeoisie. They made a lot of money. Theirs was the privilege of kissing brides whose hair they had dressed. Their names—André, François, Jacques, Léonard and Pierre—live on still by being used in the hairdressing saloons, or *salons*, of Britain.

The power of hairdressers and barbers in general was such that when, in 1776, Louis XVI set about disbanding the guilds of tradesmen, only the guild of *perruquiers-coiffeurs* remained intact: the national exchequer could not afford the huge sum of money needed for buying back the positions purchased.

One of the famous women's hairdressers was Le Gros. In 1763 he set up in the Place Vendôme, Paris, an exhibition of about thirty dolls, each with its hair arranged in a variation of one of his styles. These dolls were the forerunners of many others—most of them formed with cardboard—which were to spread fashion ideas throughout Europe.

Le Gros, having become famous, knew how to keep himself in the public eye. He created the *Académie de Coiffure*, the first regular school of hairdressing; students who completed courses there (girls as well as young men were taken) were rewarded with medals which were said to have the value of diplomas.

Models employed for demonstrations at the school had to be extremely pretty; they were known as *prêteuses de têtes*, takers of hair arrangements. When têtes prepared by students turned out well, Le Gros had the work shown off to the public by a 'prêteuse de têtes' strolling about the boulevardes. But Le Gros did not confine his talents to working with hair: he wrote a book called *L'Art de la coiffure des dames* which enjoyed wide sales despite the high price of two louis.

Le Gros's school of hairdressing was soon followed by others, all called—rather pretentiously—*académies*. The hairdressers liked the word and took to writing above their shop fronts the legend '*Académicien de coiffures et de modes*'.

This phrase was brought into being by Léonard Autier, a hairdresser who prospered under Louis XVI and became even better known than Le Gros. Hairdresser to Marie Antoinette herself, the possessor of a magnificent carriage and horses, he became known as *le grand Léonard*. One of his specialities was the art of working in scraps of chiffon, which appeared as little folds of colour among the locks of his ladies' hair.

Women's hair arrangements changed continually according to the whim of the great Léonard. He was responsible, indeed, for most of the tall and monumental styles already referred to. He emigrated to Russia during the Revolution. When he eventually returned to France in 1823, the Count of Artois found him a job as an undertaker.

The fashion for elaborate coiffures died within a few years of the French Revolution getting under way. In 1793 Louis XVI, Marie Antoinette and many other aristocrats lost their lives at the guillotine. In that year there reached England a weird fashion, inspired by these horrific events, called *la coiffure à la victime*. The natural hair was cut short and worn carefully dishevelled and wild. Some went so far in bad taste as to wear with this coiffure a crimson ribbon round the neck.

Among other short, seemingly casual styles for women was the porcupine, in which the hair on the top and front of the head was made to stand up. There was a fad, too, for

71

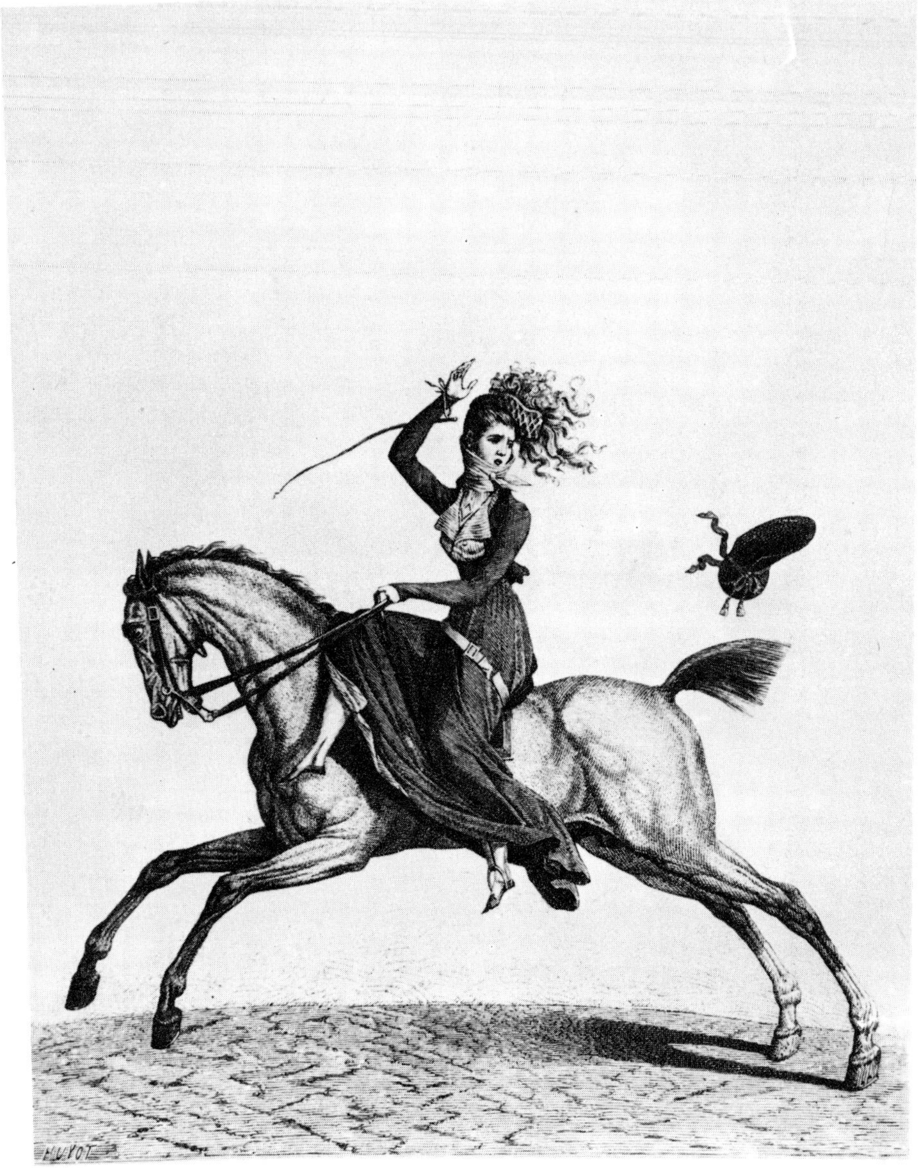

Insecure ladies' fashion wig in one of the carefully dishevelled styles, late eighteenth century. Note wide diamond mesh of foundation hair that was cut within an inch or two of the scalp; but this one did not last. Many women, indeed, bought moderate-sized wigs called cache-folies.

James Laver in *Clothes*, 1952, points out that just as women's head-dresses were prominent immediately before the French Revolution, so they were again just before the First World War when everyone wanted a cartwheel hat loaded with birds and flowers. Giving so much prominence to the female head was not only a portent, he writes; it was a protest. 'In their symbolic language they [the head-dresses] were saying something, and what they were saying was "Votes for Women". After a great social upheaval women permitted themselves very small heads as a sign that some kind of victory had been won.'

Eleven

Gentlemen's invisible perukes—nineteenth century

Men's wigs became potentially comic at the beginning of the nineteenth century when private people had taken to wearing their own hair cut very short. The professional men who still wore them—the doctors, clergymen and lawyers—were now subject to amused comment in the event of a mishap. Daniel O'Connell invited a laugh deliberately at an election meeting in Dublin in the 1830s when he lifted his wig to meet an opponent's taunt that without it his head was little to boast of.

Previously a man had thought nothing of allowing his shaved head to be seen from time to time, and if his wig came off unexpectedly he need not suppose himself a figure of fun. The wig of Frederick the Great fell off one day as he too carelessly raised his hat to the people while riding in the 1770s through Berlin. He rode on unconcerned.[37] In 1830, on the other hand, it was very embarrassing for the apothecary of Robert Seymour's drawing when he lost his wig on mounting an excitable horse. The accident was witnessed by a party of huntsmen:

> And tho' no *cry* the huntsmen *heard*,
> They saw the Doctor—*bald!*[38]

In the eighteenth century a clergyman staying at a good inn might quite naturally have handed his wig to a servant before retiring and asked him for a night cap. But it is intentionally ridiculous in *The Tours of Doctor Syntax*, published in the early nineteenth century, when Doctor

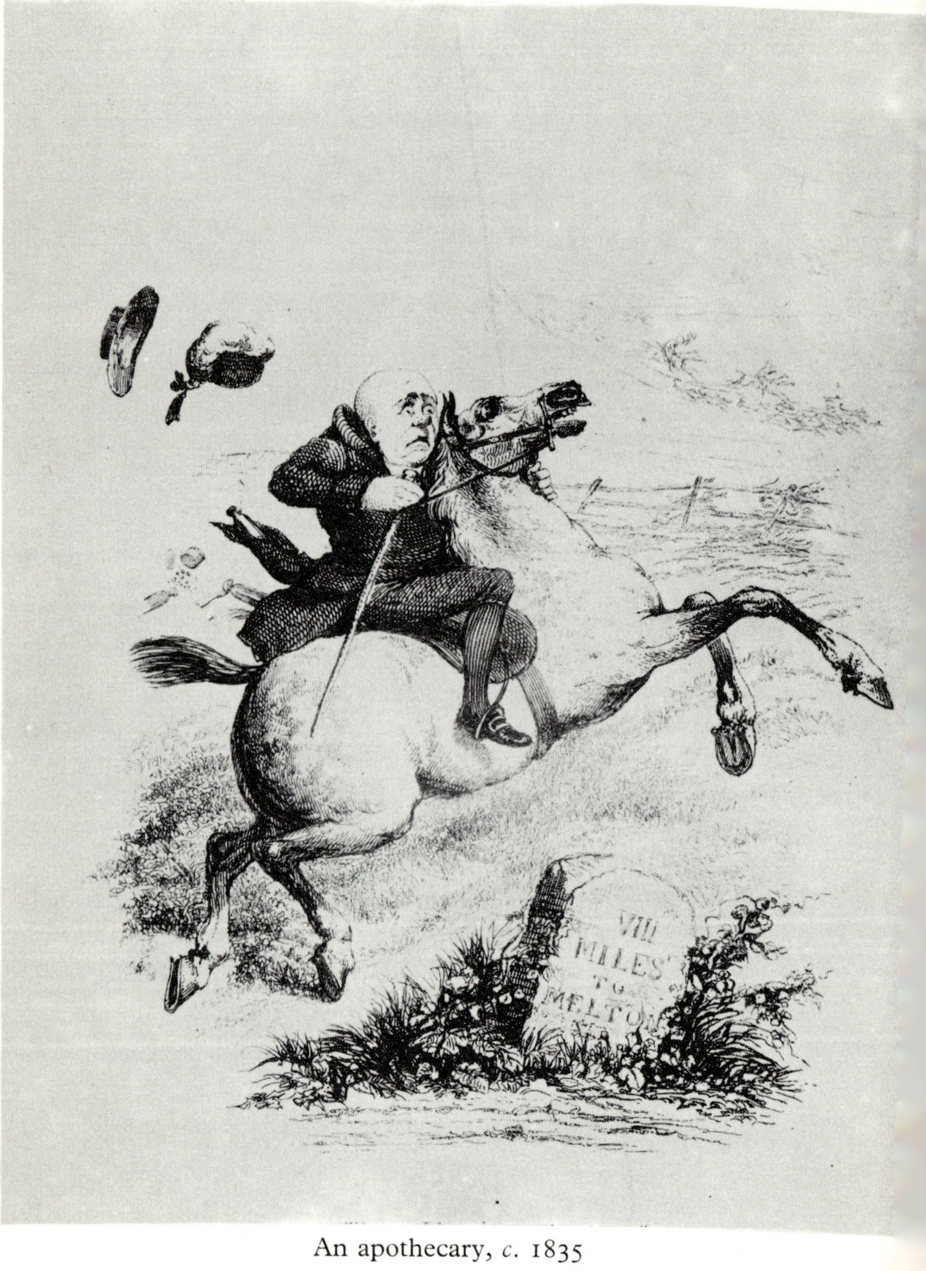

An apothecary, *c.* 1835

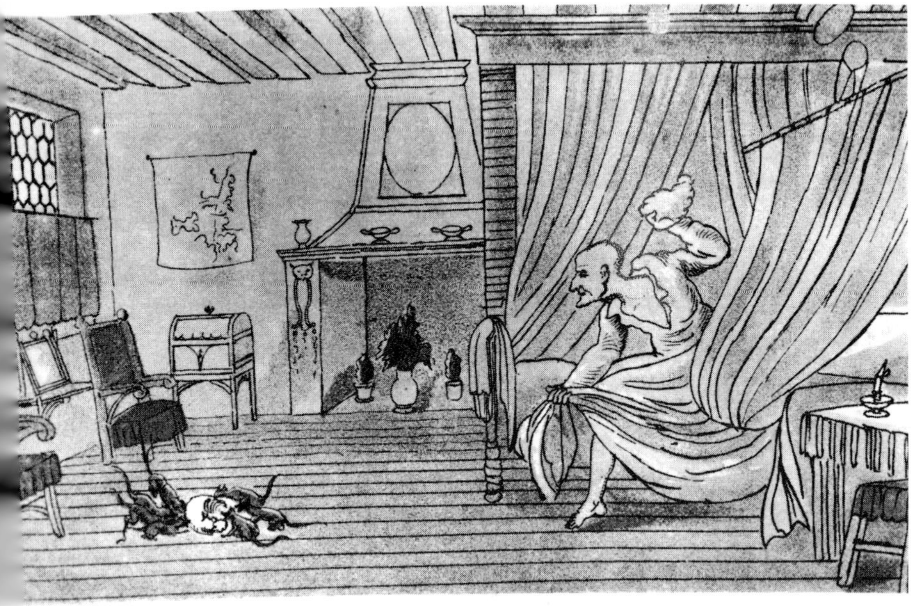

Doctor Syntax about to throw his night cap at rats mauling his wig

Syntax thus commands an inn servant:

> Go, tell the maid to shew the bed,
> Where I may lay my aching head;
> Here, take my wig, and bring a cap;
> My eyelids languish for a nap. . . .

William Combe made the most of his character's wig. It gets caught on the horns of a cow; it is dislodged when highwaymen attack him and leave him tied to a tree.

Once, during a night at an inn, he is aroused by the bustling noise of the wig being mauled by a troop of frisking rats. Having summoned the ostler to get rid of the rats, Dr Syntax goes to sleep again, not realizing until the morning that his wig has become utterly unwearable. The landlord is sent for. He enters, bowing, and offers assurances that no such complaint has ever been made before. Dr

Syntax cuts this short:

> Tell me, landlord, does your town
> A skilful peruke-maker own,
> Who can this caxon* dire restore
> To the same form it had before?

The landlord names the local barber and observes:

> I doubt not, Sire, that to a hair,
> He will your mangled wig repair.

But the man, when he arrives, declares that the wig is beyond mending; all he can do is to offer a second-hand wig. The incident closes—very amusingly for contemporary readers—with Dr Syntax continuing his journey unsuitably dressed in a two-tailed lawyer's wig.

Wigs lingered late among clergymen, who wore them at all times—that is, not just while on duty in church. Bishops were still going about in them during the Reform Bill agitations of 1831 and thereby made themselves easy targets for the mob's anger. A bishop who wore his physical bob while preaching one Sunday at St Bride's, Fleet Street, was publicly insulted. Largely as a result of this incident, all bishops gave up everyday use of the wigs which made them so conspicuous. Bishop Blomfield, Bishop of London, obtained the permission of William IV for the clergy to be wigless even when sitting as members of the episcopal bench. Archbishop Sumner was the last clergyman to wear a fashion wig; he is shown with it in a painting by John Phillip of the marriage of the Princess Royal in 1858.

It might be thought that, as a result of the disuse of male fashion wigs, the wigmakers would have been kept at least reasonably busy covering men's bald patches. But hardly anyone wanted a necessity wig. Wigs, like false teeth, were considered a shameful vanity. They were almost unmentionable; yet they were too obvious not to be immediately noticed. On the rare occasions when they were advertised

* Caxon, a weather-beaten wig

77

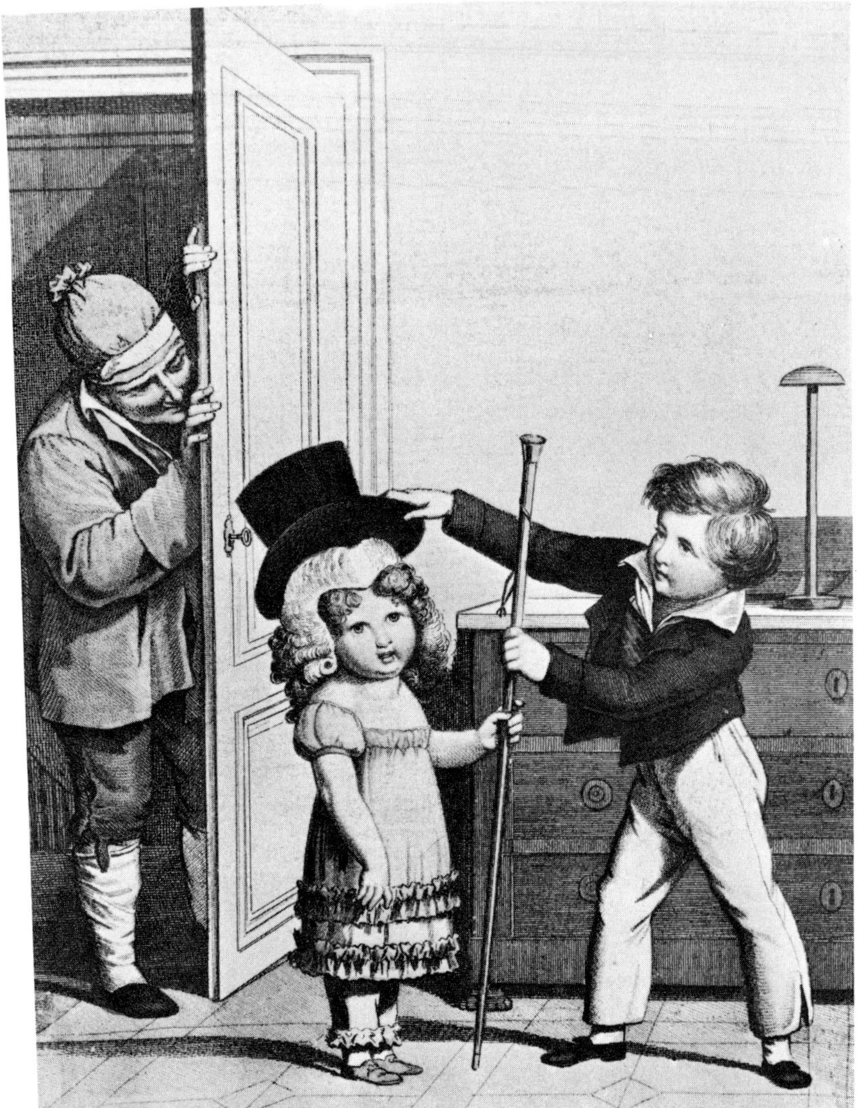

'Grand Papa's Wig', *c.* 1835. Note wig stand

in the Press, they were given a euphemism like 'gentleman's invisible peruke' or 'gentleman's head of hair'.

An advertisement of 1840 by Ross and Sons of Bishopsgate Street, London, drew attention to Invisible Ventilating Perukes,[39] and claimed that these offered 'so close a resemblance to nature as to defy detection'. The firm had 'a large assortment always kept for inspection, any one of which, if approved of, saves the purchaser time and trouble'. People wishing to order by post, without a visit, were invited to send their measurements as follows:

> Round the head in manner of a fillet, leaving the ears loose. From the forehead over to the poll, as deep each way as required. From ear to ear across the forehead, close down to the point level with the whisker.

For those interested in partial wigs the following measurements were requested:

> From the front as far forward as required to the hair behind. From one side to the other across the forehead as far as bald. Across the crown or rise of head.

Even with the small diagrams supplied, these instructions must have been hard to follow—and the fit of the resultant wig uncertain. But men who wore wigs for baldness in the nineteenth century were at least fortunate in that hair-styles were shaggy; the hair line was not expected to show (hair could hang down on the forehead) and natural-hair partings, always the weak point in a wig, were commonly rudimentary or non-existent. In theory, at least, wigs should have been less noticeable than later on, when 'short back and sides' became the custom; in practice many of them were absurdly obvious.

Aversion to wig-wearing by men seemed to grow as the Victorian period proceeded. Even the trade Press could not take men's wigs seriously. During the first thirteen years of the publication of the *Hairdressers' Weekly Journal*, founded in 1882, they were the subject of barely half a dozen edi-

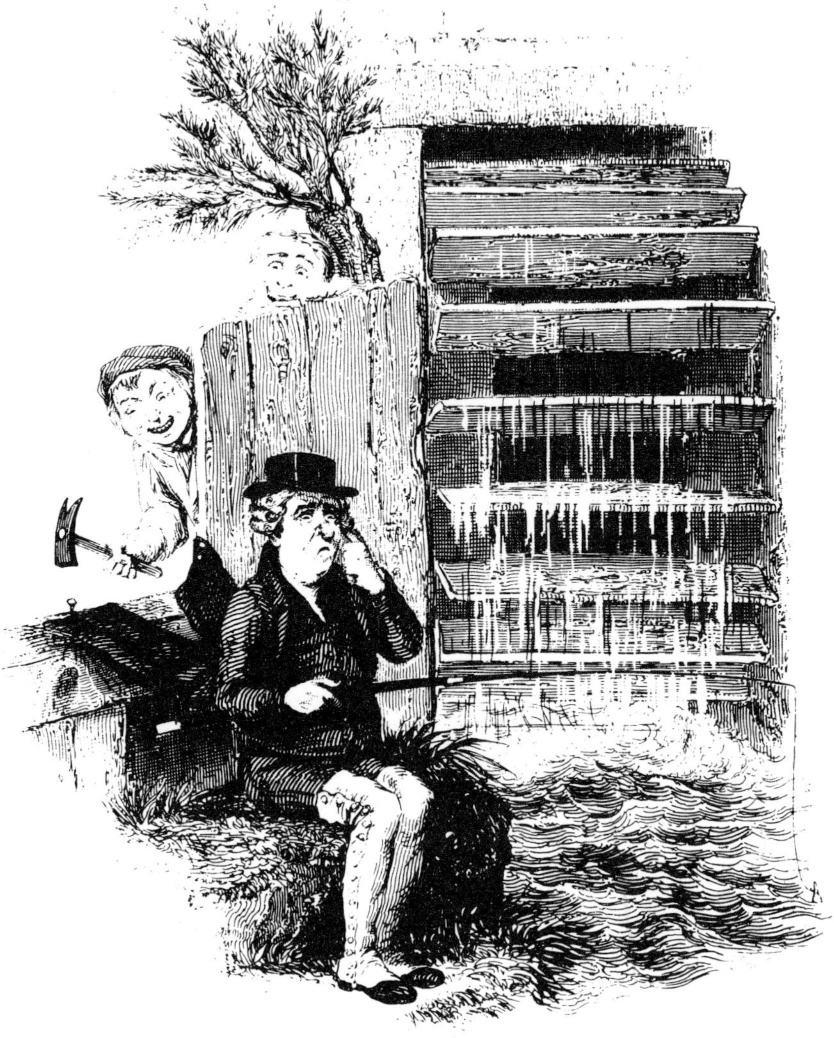

Clergyman in bob wig with three tiers of buckles. Original caption: 'This mill makes a plaguey hammering'

torial references, and all of these were either facetious or otherwise derogatory. One editorial makes fun of old men with wigs too young for them and with dyed moustaches and whiskers; another seeks to amuse with reflections about a woman's anger at finding that she cannot effectively pull the hair of a wigged husband. 'One great misfortune connected with wig-wearing', says a leading article of 1886, 'is the opportunity it affords for small boys to call out, "Hullo Wiggy! keep your hair on, old boy" '.

In 1886 the London *Evening News* summed up the situation as follows: 'Wig-wearing outside the theatrical professions is rare, though a few foolish old men, ashamed of being bald, and a few silly old maids, and often matrons, anxious to hide the footsteps of advancing age, give some employment in the manufacture of wigs, patches and fronts.'

In America meanwhile there had been great technical advances. Men could be fitted with wigs they were proud of. The greatest step forward was the introduction in New York in 1867 of fine hair lace, a net made entirely of human hair for use as a foundation material. Strips of similar material are still used for the partings of good wigs. The lace allowed the wearer's scalp to show through; and when the hairs, individually selected, were knotted to the mesh, they appeared to be growing naturally. Here was a big improvement on all previous nets for partings; a 'flesh-coloured' net which had caused a stir when introduced in France between 1805 and 1810 looked by comparison coarse.

Where expense was no object, New York wigmakers turned out superb wigs with foundations made almost wholly of hair lace. The hair could be parted anywhere, like growing hair, to give a parting which looked exactly like a parting on the natural scalp. English and French wigmakers also undertook wigs on bases of hair lace—and there is no doubt that some of them bear comparison with the best that can be made today. Records exist to show that the firm of

John Stevens of Bristol, for example, had made several wigs of this type by the year 1870: not only was the foundation entirely hair but all the sewing was done with hair. The firm's last hair-only (and incidentally springless) wig was made in 1926—for £50.

The American *Hairdresser and Perfumer* related in 1882 how a young man with a very expensive blonde, hair-lace wig was obliged to take it back to his barber. A chunk of hair was missing. He explained that a girl had asked him for a lock of his hair and he had found himself acquiescing. But the girl was gentle with him, he said, and although she cut off the lock close to the head, she did not notice that he was wearing a wig.

The barber-wigmaker would not restore the wig all at once. He spread the task over a period, imitating the natural growth by means of short pieces of hair which were exchanged from time to time for longer pieces. The girl did not find out that the young man was bald until after they were married.

By the 1890s a man with money had no great difficulty in being fitted with a brilliantly executed wig; he feared, though, society's scarcely lessened disdain for the idea of men in wigs. However, the *Hairdressers' Weekly Journal* at last, in 1895, permitted itself some hopeful remarks on the subject:

> As false teeth are now no longer a source of reproach amongst us, so universal is their use, neither will false hair in the near future tempt the finger of the scorner, so absolutely necessary will it become to most of us . . . Why should not the wigs be as recognized a necessity as false teeth or spectacles? If it were a ludicrous caricature of nature, we could understand the popular aversion to it, but this it no longer is.

The paper went on to suggest that in a changeable climate it was important for bald heads to have a covering—and what more natural than the hair which ought to be there?

The final argument in favour of 'the modern wig' was that its manufacture gave employment to a 'vast amount of female labour, all the more delicate parts being done by women'. The rosier hopes of the trade were dashed, however, in the early twentieth century, when it became the fashion for men to brush their hair straight back from the hairline.

Twelve

Ladies' imperceptible hair coverings—nineteenth century

Heads were dressed too small after the French Revolution to offer much pretext for the decorative use of false hair. Women who contrived to clip on a few curls did so with circumspection, for false hair had suddenly become associated with defects of nature. 'I wish it to be as deceiving as possible,' wrote Maria, Lady Stanley, ordering in 1802 a small 'fillet of hair for the front'; she enclosed a sample of hair and explained that the fillet was required merely because her own hair was inclined to go 'out of curl in the damp summer evenings'.

For women who had lost their hair—and hereditary female baldness was not uncommon in those days—life in the Regency period brought new and painful anxieties. Only the best posticheurs could make a short wig look natural, and classical shortness was almost the rule during the first twenty years of the nineteenth century. Sometimes the short hair was arranged in small curls all over the head and sometimes it was left straight and cut in different lengths, Titus style, to give a carefully ragged look. Brief and seemingly haphazard fringes were much favoured.

The 1820s saw the start of the long era of the neat central parting, accompanied by marked changes in women's hairstyles—changes which were less apparent in the day than in the evening. A fashion for puffs of curls at the sides of the head, and on the top, pleased the suppliers of false hair. So did the chignon, a mass of hair coiled and pinned up at the back: as the painter G. F. Watts remarked in his essay 'Taste in Dress', the taller chignons were 'mostly or always false'.

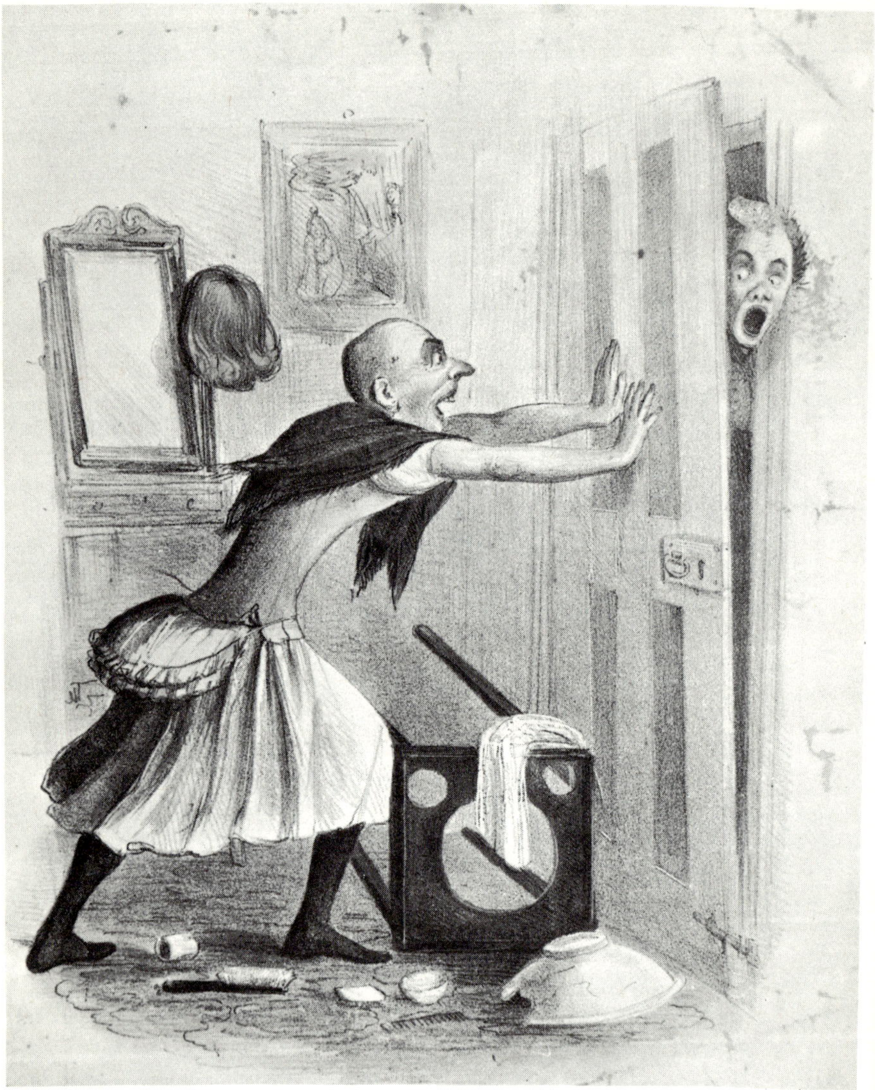

Disturbed while dressing. A print of 1840

Before long the chignon projected steeply upwards in a variety of coiling forms; it would be decorated with bird-of-paradise plumes, flowers and jewelled combs. After a lull around the middle of the nineteenth century, in which heads were flat on top, the raised-up chignon returned in the mid-1860s with even greater prominence. Small hats were worn towards the front of the head and partially supported by the chignon.

Victorian society, prudish and superficially tactful, half pretended that false hair did not exist. Rather than use the word wig, wigmakers advertised their products as 'ladies' imperceptible hair coverings'. But people liked all the same to whisper about these things, aware that quite young girls had false hair to hang at night over a bedroom chair. One of the first questions asked about a girl was:

Is it her own? through each long afternoon,
When airy muslins sweep along the grass,
Is it her own? when couples sit and spoon,
And fairy girls through tents of blossom pass,
When flower fêtes horticultural delight us,
Or promenades botanical invite us,
Then if you list you'll hear
Sweet voices whispering near,
'Is it her own?'

Is it her own? question of shelved maids
Viewing with jealous eyes their sisters fair:
Whisper of damsels whose concocted braids
Pass for luxurious wealth of golden hair:
See in sly corners dowagers conspiring,
Pleasantly smiling, audibly admiring.
Hear how their voices sink,
'Quite so; but do you think
It is her own?'[40]

In England *The Times* reported that the import of chignons from France in the year 1865 was 11,954 and that

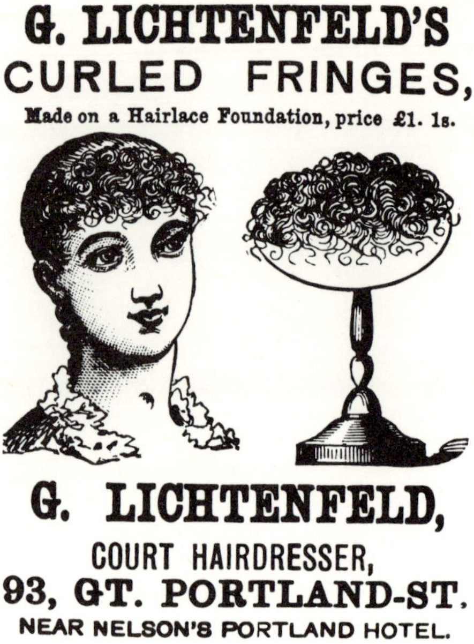

A typical advertisement of 1881

along with them came enough human hair for some 7,000 chignons to be made up in England. The value of the hair and chignons exported from France in that year was over £45,000. England, it was stated, took the largest quantity, the United States the second largest. Other hairpieces commonly used were the marteau, a flat tail of hair for pinning on at the back; the tail or switch; and the bandeau, a band of carefully dressed hair for the front which could be combed back with the growing hair.

Men often claimed to be scornful about the use of false hair. A certain Coelebs Smith wrote to London's *Punch* pointing out that a young lady who caught a husband with such a snare was guilty of obtaining matrimony by false pretences. 'Conceive', he said, 'the horror of a husband at finding that his wife took her hair off every night, together with her ear-rings . . . this is really what is meant by the wearing of a chignon.'[41] But it is likely that, once married,

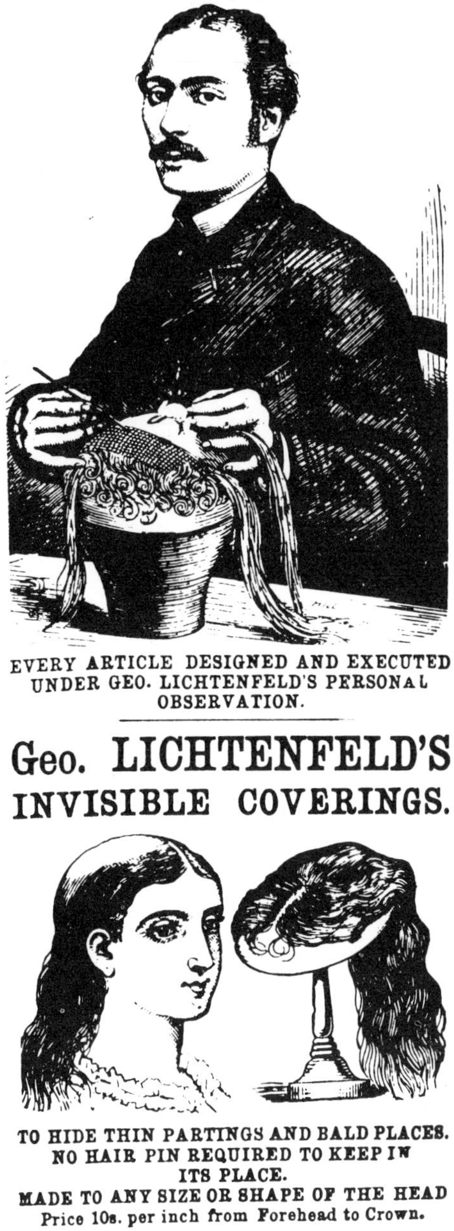

A typical advertisement of 1891. No reference to 'wigs'

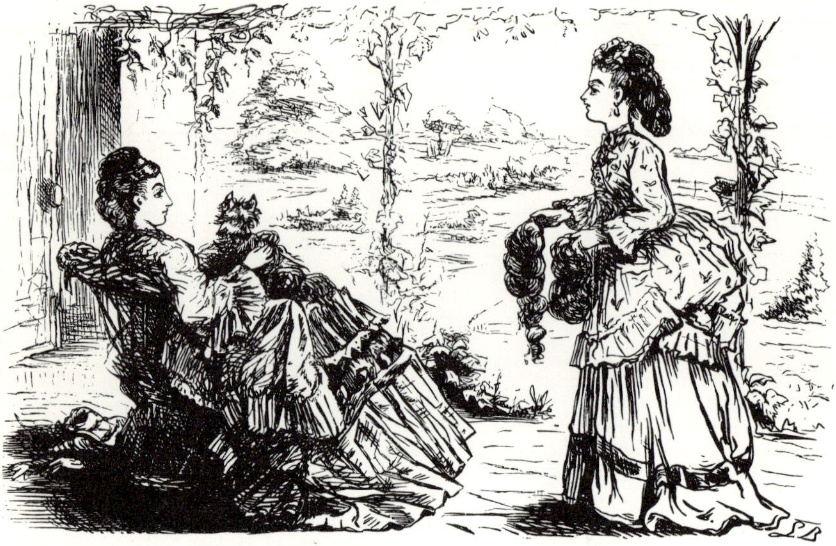

NEGLECTED GENIUS

Mistress. "No Opportunity of Improving yourself here, Parker? Why not?"
Maid. "Well, Ma'am, Ive arranged this Hair differently every Day for a Week; but as you have never put it on, and have taken to Wearing your Own, I feel as my Feelin's is hurt, and my Edication is wasted."

Cartoon from *Punch*, 1873

most men were willing allies in these modest, fashion-dictated deceptions.

A few husbands were themselves deceived by fake hair, however, so brilliant was the execution of the best hair-pieces. In the reminiscences of a retired wigmaker, whose father also was a wigmaker, there is the story of a woman with a full wig who contrived permanently to conceal the fact from her husband.

His story, offered here as true, is that a certain businessman in a provincial city, rich and no longer young, made no secret at his regular pub of an obsessive liking for girls with yellow hair which hung just below the hips. The landlady of the place had a pretty daughter with short brown hair and took the calculated step of having her fitted with an expensive wig: it was of yellow hair which fell just below the girl's hips. The businessman, seeing her behind the bar, did all

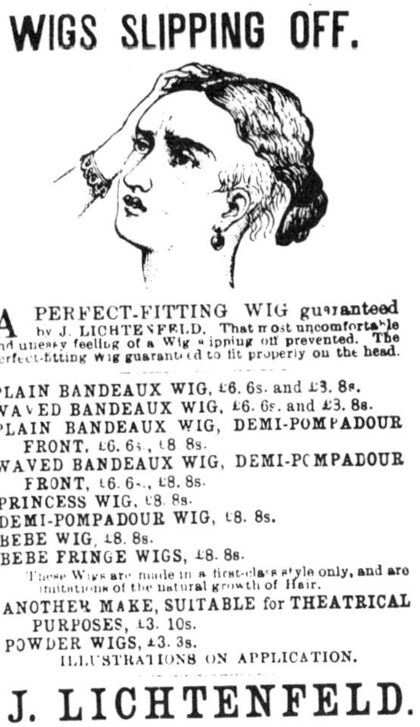

Unusual shock advertisement of 1882

the landlady hoped; he married her and was able every night to comb and fondle the wonderful long hair.

The young wife, whose head was shaved of its own hair, never removed the wig except at her wigmaker's, and her husband always admired its colour and length. It so happended that he died first; but had it been otherwise, the wife had arranged, to spare him a shock, that the wigmaker should come at once when she died and dress the hair in the coffin.

Women's hairdressers and wigmakers were accustomed to keeping secrets. If a customer wore a wig because she was bald, it was customary for no one but her own hairdresser to see her without it. Even the hairdresser's assistant would not be allowed in the room.

There was a sad reason why women of former times, including Edwardian times, were especially anxious that no

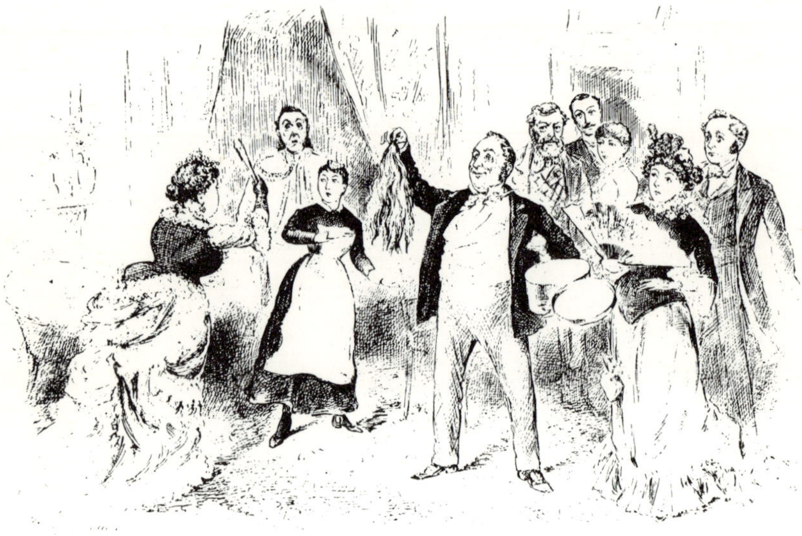

SCENE FROM "GAMMON" AT THE VAUDEVILLE

Our picture is from the last scene of Mr. Mortimer's amusing comedy. All the characters are shown, the incident being the discovery by Mr. Potts of the false hair from Truefit's for Mrs. Potts behoof. Mrs. Potts indignation with the maid Lucinda, who has been the cause of the exposé before the Sweetmans, is one of the details of the situation.

Cartoon from *Illustrated Sporting and Dramatic News*, 1882

one should think them bald: feminine baldness, it was commonly understood, meant that a parent or grandparent had contracted syphilis. In 1888 an elderly American woman caused a mild sensation when she removed her wig during a hearing at the Westminster County Court. She was defending, successfully, non-payment of a bill for a wig on the ground that it was grey instead of white as ordered. By removing the wig she had on, and pointing to what remained of her own hair, she was able to show the judge, to his embarrassment, what she meant by white.

The danger of false hair coming off inadvertently was minimized by the habit of erect posture instilled in the Victorian girl; a favourite training exercise was walking with a book balanced on the head. When an accident did occur, it was generally the result of relying less on a good fit and properly adjusted springs than on adhesives which could melt. In an unusually graphic wigs advertisement for 1882, published in England in the *Queen*, a jewelled lady who is perhaps at dinner clutches at a wig which has broken away from one side of her head. She is seen to be almost entirely bald.

In the last years of the nineteenth century there was a big decline in the amount of false hair used for a purely decorative purpose. From then until at least 1914 the main business of the wigmaker was to supply wigs for women with severe baldness.

Thirteen

Modern wigs

Except to hide baldness, false hair has been used sparingly in the twentieth century until the late 1940s. Mention must be made, though, of a feminine craze between the wars for artificial hunting buns sewn to the backs of bowler hats to prevent shingled women looking bare at the neck.

After the Second World War there was a fad for pin-on clusters of hair; and in Britain the National Health Service, which took psychological troubles into account, encouraged both men and women with unsatisfactory hair to consider procuring a wig. In the 1950s the American introduction of synthetic hair led to much experiment with fashion wigs and to their becoming accepted—first in America and then in Britain—as part of a normal wardrobe. In the 1960s most women were choosing hair of a colour to match their own; they wished people to suppose the wig a glamorous arrangement of their natural hair.

But the cheap machine-made wigs at between £3 and £20 ($8 to $50) however decorative, have rarely given this impression. They are made of wefts—that is, bands of woven hair—which are stitched one above the other on a foundation of coarse netting; to give even a semblance of nature they must have a fringe all round; they cannot be convincingly parted, and if the hairs are disarranged by handling or wind, bare patches of net are exposed. These wigs are on sale to men as well as women (the Unisex wig is designed to suit both), and are often known as fun wigs. Hairdressers call them hair hats, which seems a fair description. They can be bought off the peg at wig boutiques and at the wig counters in the big stores; the fit need not be more than approximate as they can be kept on with an elastic band.

The handmade bespoke article, which may cost between £80 and £200 ($240–600), falls into a different category: women's styles can easily go entirely undetected. The wigmaker takes seven or more measurements of a client's head, builds up a head-shaped block to the right size (it is labelled with the client's name), then mounts the braid and fine net foundation which is to receive the hair.

The hairs need not all go in singly, though some wigmakers will attach no more than three at a time; the most important provision for a lifelike head of hair is the careful mixing of two or three related shades (where dyed natural hair is obvious, the explanation is that all hairs are of the same colour).

Over the greater part of the wig the hairs are knotted with a special needle on the net foundation. In the area of the parting, where the foundation consists of almost invisible lace or parting silk, the hairs are inserted one or two at a time and drawn through—that is, the knot is on the underside. This is one of the main tricks in making a wig look natural: once firmly in place on the head, the natural scalp shows through the fine lace and the hairs appear to be growing from it. When the line of scalp revealed by a parting has to be artificially suggested, wigmakers have often made the mistake of inserting a strip of foundation material which is pink. On a normally hirsute head the scalp shows through white rather than pink. For a first-class full wig between 50,000 and 150,000 hairs are needed, according to texture, but a neat-fingered operator—probably a girl who has served a four-year apprenticeship—can finish the job in a week.

Women's wigs of a high order of craftsmanship have been available, for people of means anyway, since the early nineteenth century; but it must be said that pinch-pleated styles did nothing to help them look natural. Today even moderately-priced fashion wigs can be good enough for everyday use. Men's wigs of necessity continue to be very difficult to make natural-looking. Often they do not look natural even in the photographs used for advertisements. But if the style is to include hair combed away from the forehead, a satisfactory appearance can be achieved only by skilled work with a strip of fine lace. Through this lace hairs of different lengths are individually drawn and knotted, and irregularly spaced. For an article worn every day there is the drawback, however, that a lace-fronted wig may take as much as half an hour to adjust; and from time to time it is necessary to trim the lace with scissors to stop it looking frayed.

It can certainly be a help to the conscientious wigmaker if his client has hair of his own above the ears and at the back, but great pains must be taken to ensure that the false hair matches this exactly in colour and texture, and that it will not change in appearance in strong sunlight or after being out in a shower of rain. Needless to say, it must fit the scalp perfectly and not shift. Flat tension springs sewn into the neck of a full wig hold it tightly on the head without assistance from adhesives.

Several new ways of making men's necessity wigs have been put into practice since 1964—though without making them much less detectable. The bases are no longer invariably of net (whether hair, silk, cotton or nylon): it is now possible to have a wig with the hairs implanted in a base of a flexible plastic material, or of fibreglass which is solid rather than flexible. Both types are prepared with the aid of a cast of the head.

An early experimenter with solid-based wigs was Mr Reginald Dooley, a bald man exasperated by the nuisance of having to use spirit for cleaning his wig. On 13 February 1969 he dived in a wig of this type from a swimming pool's twelve-metre board, and had himself photographed in the air, hitting the water and surfacing. There can be no doubt, from the photographs, that the wig stayed in position; and

Mr Dooley's claim that it was not spoiled by the water is supported by the experiences of other wearers. But perhaps the best selling point of these rigid-based wigs is that the hairs are so firmly anchored that they can be washed in hot soapy water; this is the one treatment which wearers of traditional wigs have to avoid, since water tends to loosen hairs knotted to a net. Retention, aided by sticky tapes, is limpet-like. A Dooley wig will stay on the head even if directly pulled. Indeed it is not too easy for the wearer himself to remove such a wig; he may have to use a comb or a shoehorn to start the process of levering it upwards from the back.

Another type of men's wig is fastened to the head by having the existing hair woven through the net base. This is sometimes known as interlinking. The result may appear natural enough, but a wig which cannot be removed at night will sooner or later cause irritation. There is also the disadvantage that as the natural hair grows, usually half an inch a month, the wig becomes progressively looser on the scalp. The makers recommend a return visit once every four or five weeks for tightening; but a client in Britain reported to the Consumers' Association in 1969 that he had found the wig too uncomfortable to continue wearing it after ten days. He stated that it had cost him £150 (about $450) and taken two hours to fit: periodic re-weavings were to cost him between £5 and £10 ($15–30) a time.

This wig-wearer was one of 196 who co-operated in a survey conducted by *Which?* the magazine of the Consumers' Association; over half of them, incidentally, were under forty years old and one in six was under thirty. The resultant report tabulated useful information and opinion about the various brands of wig to be had in 1969 and also tried to explain why bald men wished to hide, with an artifice which could be most exacting, a condition which in men is socially acceptable and sometimes positively distinguished.

Three-quarters of the number said it was because a wig

made them look younger, or made them look the age they thought they would have looked but for their loss of hair. Half said a wig gave them more confidence, and rather more than half claimed that it kept the head warm and protected it from knocks.

The alleged disadvantages of wearing a wig of necessity were also summarized in the article in *Which?* It was said that once a man had appeared in a wig, and had it accepted by some as his natural hair, he could not easily appear without it; he was therefore committed to the continual expense of sticking plasters (essential for toupees or partials) and of professional maintenance—and also of buying at least one spare wig. Wigs were inclined, it was noted, to fade or change colour in sunlight; they could be hot to wear; healthy sweating through the scalp allowed them to become unstuck. They were disarranged awkwardly by wind, and had to be covered if exposed to rain or snow. Some of those who took part in the survey warned bald men to beware of the sort of wig which made them look younger than their wives; elderly men considering a wig were reminded that a thick and bushy one could look incongruous.

Clearly a lot of men feel furtive about their wigs; they have an irrational, perhaps subconscious, fear that they could be suddenly dislodged. There have thus been people prepared to pay enormous sums on transplant operations. In these, chunks of scalp and growing hair are taken from the sides and back of the head and made to grow on the bald patch. Frank Sinatra, it was reported early in 1970, invested £4,000 (about $12,000) in a hair-by-hair transplant.

To secure the wigs of totally bald men, a Boston hairdresser has actually had a few customers fitted with anchor points in the form of steel loops let into the scalp.

Fourteen

Legal wigs

> Who would have supposed that this grotesque ornament, fit only for an African chief, would be considered indispensably necessary for the administration of justice in the middle of the nineteenth century?
>
> John Campbell,
> *The Lives of the Lord Chancellors*, 1845

The legal wig is still considered necessary in England well after the middle of the twentieth century. Few would deny that it has a levelling and dignifying effect on the barristers, differing widely in personal appearance, who plead in the courts.

Obviously, to avoid ridicule, the wig must be always neat and managed with circumspection, and never sit even half an inch askew. Mismanagement can create an anecdote which never dies. Lawyers still refer to a classic incident of

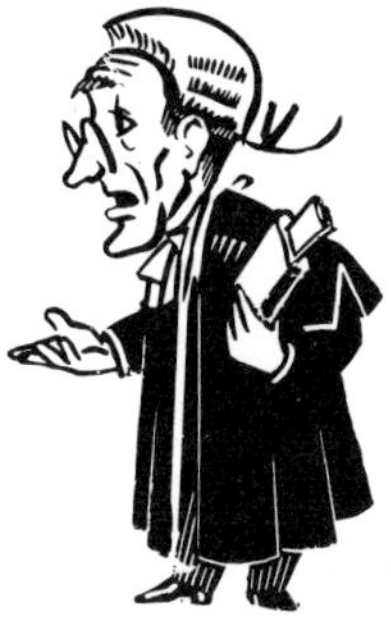

Barrister in wig and gown

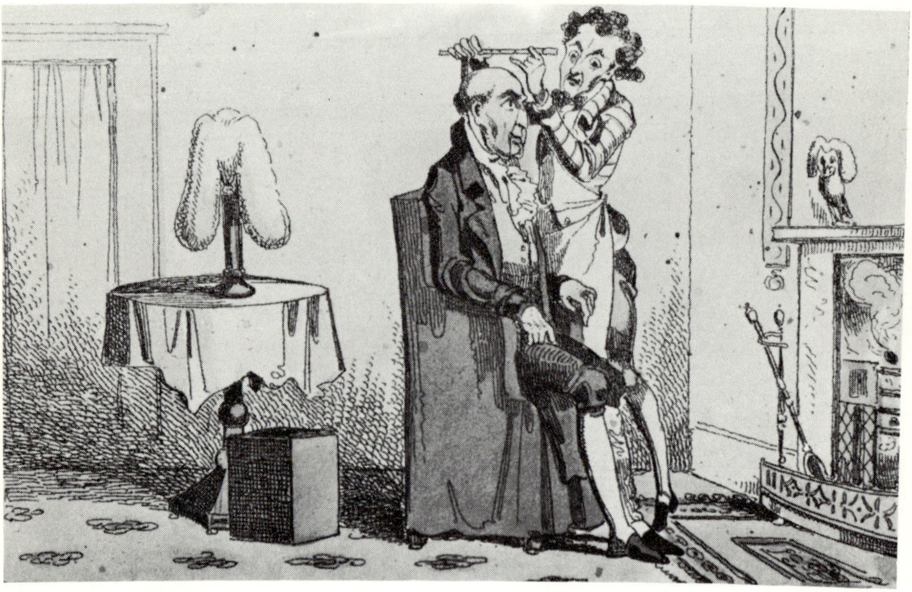

Judge being measured for a new long-bottom, 1823.
Original caption: 'Bless me, what a long head you've got, my Lord. Well, I declare tis as thick as it's long.'

the late nineteenth century concerning a judge in full dress attending an assizes service in Oxford. Dr Lang, long before he became Archbishop of Canterbury, was preaching the sermon and had decided on a text illustrating the importance of respect for authority. He chose 'Go up thou bald head', taken from the story in the Book of Kings in which Eliseus is mocked. Unfortunately, as the judge entered the church—when it was too late to alter the sermon—his wig caught on a projection over the doorway, and remained for a moment suspended, revealing that he was as bald as an egg.[42]

The barrister is in a stupid situation if he finds, just before going into court, that a joker has tampered with the set of his wig. This eventuality is considered in a mid-nineteenth-century patent for a forensic wig; it was said to be constructed on a principle which prevented the curls being mauled and 'the possibility of any person untying the tails'.

All men feel a little different on putting on a wig, and it does appear that the legal kind, grotesque or not, beneficially affects performance. It used to be said of the famous Scottish lawyer, Lord Erskine (1746–1817), that he was a strange contrast in and out of his wig and gown. Out of it he talked in a gauche and almost foolish way; but in it he could persuade people to entrust their lives to his hands. Charles James Fox recounted how Erskine, when not in his wig, had replied to a question put to him while the two were on a council of the cabinet. 'Oh yes,' he said, 'depend upon it, it must be so, for I remember it was in an old Presbyterian book of prophecies which my mother had.'[43]

The barrister's wig is traditionally of fine white horsehair with thirty curls. According to the researches of James Derriman (*Pageantry of the Law*, 1955), wigs came into use by barristers only gradually; some of the judges, though wearing full-bottom wigs themselves, considered the large wigs so 'coxcombical' on lesser lawyers that they would not allow young members of the bar to plead in them. It is doubtful if the long curled periwig fashionable in the reigns of Charles II and James II ever became generally adopted by barristers while at work.

During the reign of William and Mary, senior lawyers devoted much attention to rules for dress and appearance. To check the display of long beards, which was worrying some of them, an order was issued by the Inner Temple that no member 'should wear his beard above three weeks' growth on pain of forfeiting 20s'. The Middle Temple ordered that no member 'should wear great breeches in their hose, made after the Dutch, Spanish or Almain fashion, or lawn upon their caps, or cut doublets, under a penalty of 3s 4d, and expulsion for the second offence'. All four Inns of Court forbade, for any but 'knights and benchers', the wearing of a velvet cap, velvet shoes, a scarf, double shirt cuffs and feathers or ribbons on the head. The adoption of the wig was to solve the headgear problem. Today members of the Inns of Court dine in hall bareheaded.

It was certainly the custom, later in the first quarter of the eighteenth century, for all barristers to wear wigs; but they wore the more convenient short type with tightly arranged curls, the type which was becoming fashionable among private gentlemen. In its final form, the barrister's wig is technically a combination of the tye wig and the Ramillies. Up to the early nineteenth century it was rather fuller than at present and powdered.

Some barristers ceased to powder their wigs around 1830 with the introduction of wigs which simulated the powder finish. Croake James relates that Justice Allan Park resisted the change as an innovation in the constitution, and actually refused to recognize his own son when he appeared at the bar in one of the new powderless, hygienic wigs. But such is the conservatism of the bar that powdered wigs continued to be worn on the Oxford circuit far into the nineteenth century. George Bancroft, Clerk of Assize on the Midland Circuit, who retired in 1946, was still wearing a powdered wig in 1939.[44]

A rule made by the judges in Britain in March 1922—just before the first woman was called to the bar—lays down that women are to wear wigs 'which shall completely cover and conceal the hair'. It is reported that, during the meeting which drew up this rule, two of the judges—Darling and Horridge—proposed that women should wear instead the biretta, which is a square cap; but the idea was disapproved of by the other nine judges present.

The full-bottom wig of judges and Queen's Counsel, adopted in the 1660s because it was the correct everyday fashion for gentlemen, remains (as stated in Chapter 6) part of the ceremonial dress for state occasions. It consists in its modern form of a curled or frizzed crown with long flaps; these flaps have twenty or more rows of curls made from the manes of horses. State occasions for wearing it may include meals: at the Lord Mayor's Day banquet in London, and at the pre-assizes official breakfast at York, the judges in their full-bottom wigs do not always find it easy to eat gracefully. Until about 1850 this large type of wig was worn by judges not only on state occasions but also when trying any kind of alleged crime.

For day-to-day wear on the bench judges have since then used a short tye wig. This differs from the barrister's wig in that it has only one curl, a vertical curl just over the queue. A small bare patch on the crown of a judge's wig is a reminder of the times, before wigs became a fashion, when judges wore the coif, a close-fitting black cloth cap. On the coming of wigs as normal wear, a hole was left in the judge's wig to allow the coif to be seen. It was at that time still worn beneath the wig.

The main change in legal wigs during the past 170 years has been a gradual reduction in size, particularly in the tye wig and the barrister's curled wig. Both of these were much bushier in the early 1800s, and judges wearing their full-bottoms, as was the custom in society and among men who had abandoned wigs, often felt tiresomely conspicuous. Lord Eldon, an early-nineteenth-century Lord Chancellor, decided to seek permission from the king to appear with his own hair when not sitting in court. According to Croake James, who writes that Eldon made the request to please his wife, he pointed out to the king (whether George III or George IV is not stated) that 'so lately as the reigns of James I and Charles I judicial wigs were unknown'. 'True,' replied the king, 'I admit the correctness of your statement and am willing, if you like it, that you should do as they did; for though they certainly had no wigs, yet they wore long beards.'

Fifteen

Where the hair comes from

> The hour of bitter distress was the time of his harvest, and whenever penury knocked at the door, Jock was sure to follow, if there were any fair females within . . . Often has Jock shorn the locks of a village beauty, which . . . she has at length sacrificed, with many a smothered sob and bitter tear.
>
> William Clarke, 'The Hair Pedlar', published in *The Companion to a Cigar*, 1850

Jock Macleod was a hair pedlar in Devon. To write about him in the melancholy tones then fashionable, William Clarke secretly followed him about. The gathering of human hair has always tended to be a haphazard and sometimes a sad exercise. Today British wigmakers rely for supplies on recognized hair merchants, but the hair pedlars, or hair collectors, are still in business, sending hair to the big wholesale houses who prepare it for use. They are no longer met with in the villages of Britain, but are familiar figures in Asia and in parts of Europe where peasants are ready to make a cash crop of their hair. In Italy there are still brides who raise money in this way for a dowry.

The money to be made from selling a head of hair need no longer be trifling, since it is widely known that for wigs worn daily nothing has been found to beat it. Synthetic hair, such as nylon, shines too much or too little and is uncomfortably non-absorbent; mohair, from the Angora goat, can be dressed easily but is too soft for regular wear, while the virtue of yak hair is simply its great length.

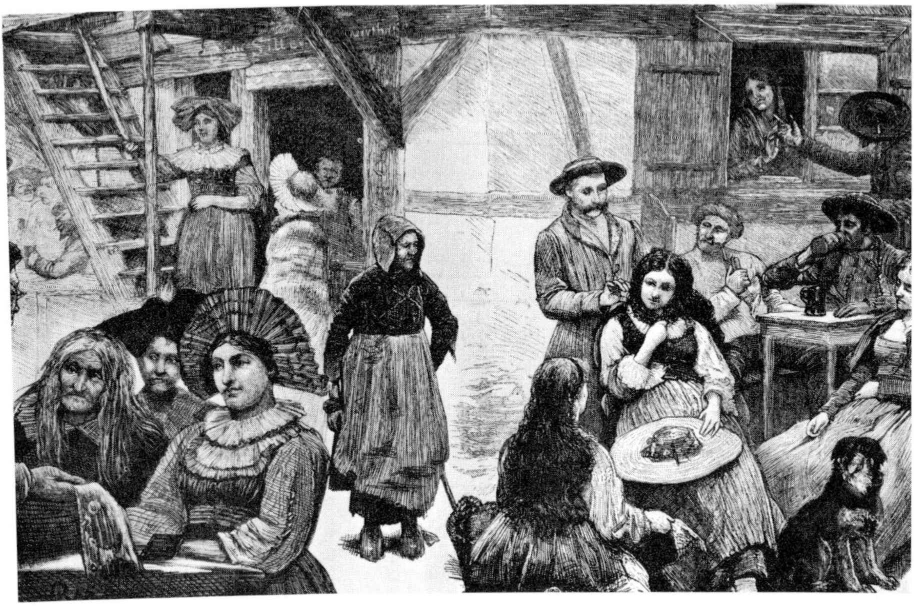

Human hair market in Alsace, 1871

Natural white hair has always been the most valuable kind; today the price to the wigmaker is about £240 ($770) a pound for the best grades. Any old lady with good white hair could, if she wished, make a handsome sum by selling part of it. In the earlier part of the twentieth century, when wigmaking was carried on locally, the master wigmaker of a town would prudently form friendly contact with old ladies in almshouses. With growth at the rate of half an inch a month, he could hope to buy a crop of white hair from each lady every two years or so. The hair from one head would usually be enough for two wigs.

Not everyone, however, can grow perfectly white hair. Denis Diderot set out the facts 200 years ago in his *Encyclopédie*:

> It is usually persons having the blackest hair whose hair eventually turns agate white. A mere pearl white is the colour which chestnut hair eventually becomes;

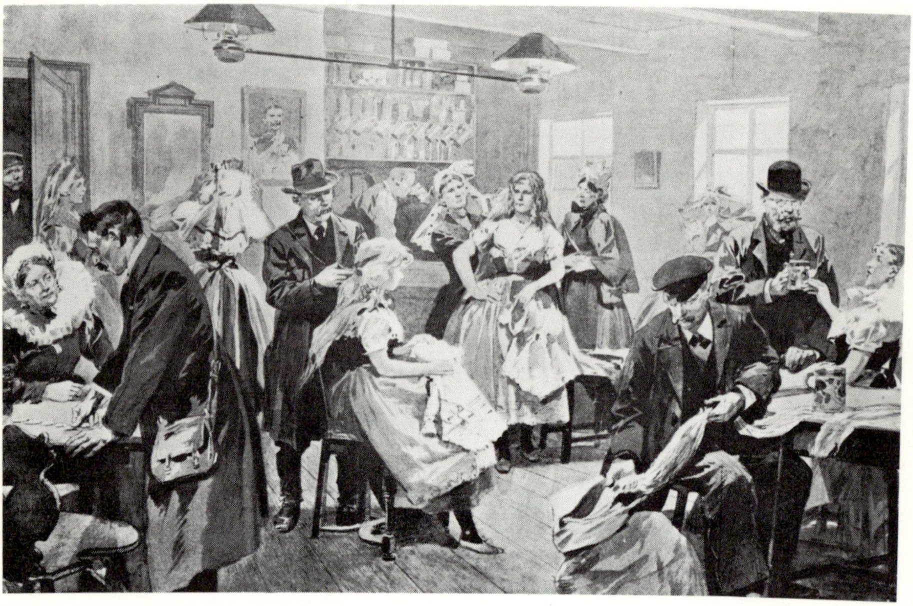

Human hair collectors with reluctant suppliers in a Berlin café, 1902

often the tips of the hair are yellow. Hair which has been fair is not such good quality as that which has been red. The body remains in red hair; it is very strong and the ends remain firm and curl naturally. This hair is without price . . . with persons having fair hair, the more they advance in age, the more their hair takes on a brownish tint and is in consequence worth less. With others the contrary is the case. As they whiten with advancing years, the more their hair improves in vigour.

After white hair, naturally blonde and reddish hair are the most expensive and, as in Roman times, much of it comes from Germany. Blonde hair is also collected in Scandinavia. The best quality dark hair comes from Spain and northern Italy, especially from Tuscany (the American firm Lisa Wigs and Wiglets specialize in hair-pieces of hair from southern Italy), while excellent brown and auburn hair comes from France. These are the types of hair needed for wigs worn regularly and for the more convincing fashion wigs.

For hair hats and cheap theatrical wigs, Asian hair is imported by the ton. It can be boiled and bleached and re-coloured, but it looks coarse beside European hair and cannot, after the chemical treatment, last as long. For the American wig firms, the greatest source of supply is Indonesia.

Until the middle of the nineteenth century much of the hair needed by wigmakers was obtained in Britain, though by no means the majority: in the *Tradesman's Universal Director* for 1753, for example, a hair merchant is described as one who both imports hair and employs people to collect it in England. In 1872 a London hair merchant was advertising in the *Hairdressers' Chronicle* a large stock of Dutch hair, claimed to be 'the finest and purest in Europe'.

In the days before collection of hair was organized to some extent, it was often stolen, or at least removed without consent—and not only, it appears, by rough pedlars. P. Stubbes, writing in 1583—at the height of a female craze for wigs—said that fashion-mad women were so anxious to obtain false hair that it was dangerous to let a child with a good head of hair wander out of sight, as sometimes women would entice such a child to a quiet place and there cut off its hair. The demand for human hair must have been considerable in 1700. Mr Stevens Cox has found a record relating to that year in which a girl is paid £60 for her hair and an old woman £50 for her grey hair.

In eighteenth-century London it was not uncommon for complete wigs, as well as locks of hair, to be stolen. Wigs of almost any kind were valuable to barbers. The wig stealer operated in crowded streets, carrying on his shoulders a small boy—even concealed there in a basket—whose job it was to seize wigs from the heads of gentlemen as they passed by. The latter were usually inhibited from making much fuss by the slightly ridiculous figures they presented with their white, shaven heads.

Customers for wigs sometimes procured the hair themselves and took it to the barber to be made up. A record of a private deal appears in the *Stapleton Archives* for 1668.[45]

> Paid to Peg Heavisides for her head of haire which I got off her towards making me a periwig, but it was too short, 2s 6d.

Margaret de Valois, wife of Henry IV of France (1553–1610), is reported to have had a wig constructed from her own hair.

Samuel Pepys supplied the barber with long hair from his own head when he first decided to become a wig-wearer. He was only thirty-one at the time and could probably offer hair that was of good quality. Usually the wigmakers preferred women's hair to men's. The hair of countrywomen, which had never been powdered, was thought especially satisfactory. Diderot maintains that 'the hair of prostitutes and of men who give way to debauchery with women dries and loses its quality.'

> But in countries where beer and cider are the common beverages, the hair is better than elsewhere. The Flemish have excellent hair; the beer nourishes and oils it. These people are nearly all either blond or light chestnut. With a little experience their hair can be easily distinguished. It becomes lighter with boiling, whereas fair hair from other countries becomes brownish.

Although reputedly inferior in quality, hair from the dead, cadaver hair, was often made use of from the sixteenth to the early nineteenth century. Shakespeare has referred to it more than once—'those crisped, snaky, golden locks . . . often known to be the dowry of a second head, the skull that bred them in the sepulchre'. 'Dead hair', the artful Jock Macleod would say, 'is of no value scarcely, for it will not hold the curl of the frizeur.' Nevertheless, he made a point of visiting cottages in which a bereavement had just taken place: he was always glad, he said, to lend a helping hand to the distressed.

France, birthplace of the fashion wig, was the first country in which the collection of human hair for wigmaking became a widespread business, giving work to hundreds of pedlars. Early in the seventeenth century these pedlars were finding they could do business best in those parts where the people habitually hid their heads beneath bonnets; at fairs in Brittany, Normandy, Beaucaire and the Auvergne they would announce themselves by calling out 'Piou Piou' ('Hair Hair') and by banging on a drum. For obvious reasons, they made their visits at regular intervals.

Peasants who were prepared to sell their hair would present themselves at the gateway or tent announced for the cutting. Mothers led forward their offspring; and the long tresses of the young girls fell one after another under the scissors of the pedlar. Often payment consisted of no more than some knick-knack or remnant of cloth or part of a bonnet. The wigmakers paid the collectors highly, on the other hand, for the hair so cheaply acquired. They all wanted hair from France; hair from hotter countries had a bad reputation. The fact that they were using great quantities of hair from horses and goats was an indication of short supply of human hair.

By the end of the seventeenth century purchases of hair took place in England at town and country fairs. The hair pedlar looked about for women and girls suitably equipped; then approached them with flattering remarks and set about bargaining. Directly a sale was agreed, the pedlar cut off the hair as close to the scalp as the agreement permitted, bound the root ends together and put the bundle in his collecting sack. He had what was called a head of hair.

Sometimes the pedlar wielded his scissors before a sale was properly agreed. Jock Macleod was 'wily in his bargains beyond credence'. He sometimes managed to cut off the locks of a young girl before a definite price had been fixed.

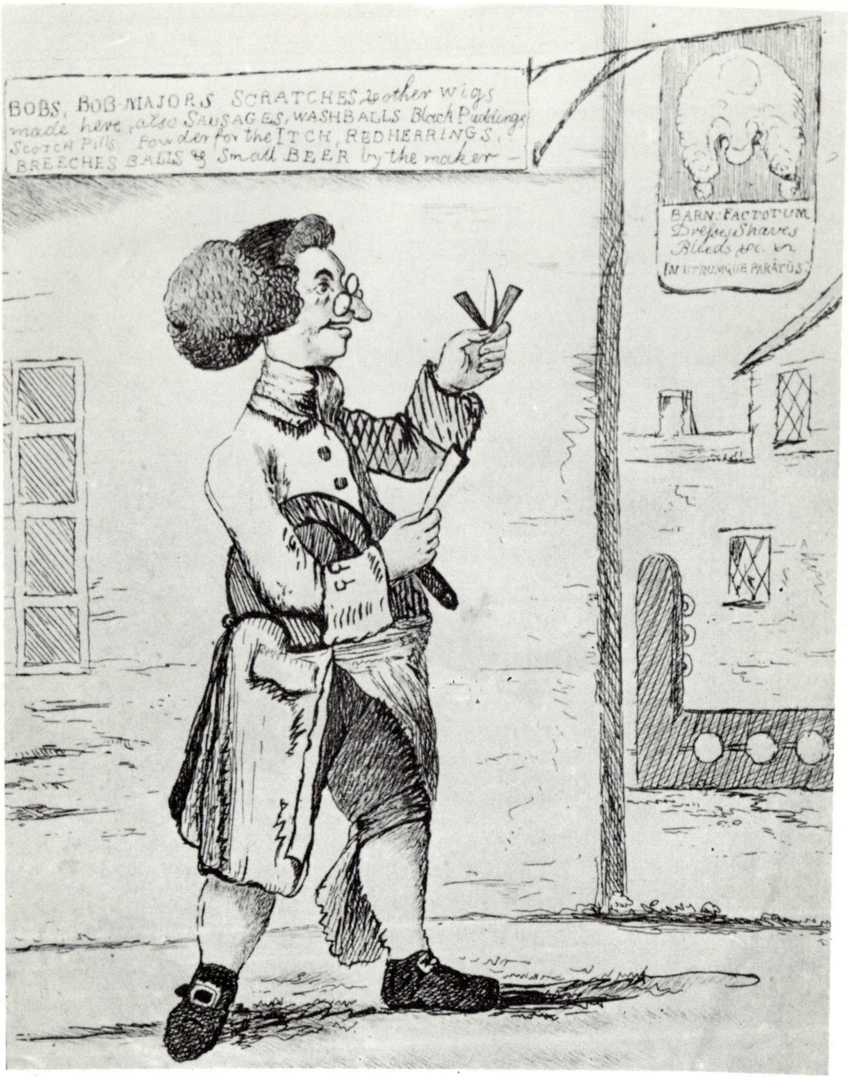

Village barber, 1772. Barbers as well as cartoonists could be jocular about their services. An eighteenth-century Lewes barber had on his signboard a picture of Absalom caught by his hair in the branches of an oak, and below it this couplet:

Oh, Absalom, unlucky prig,
why didst not wear a periwig?

He then poised it in his hand and effected wonder at its being so much less than he had expected. Working it with his fingers, he would pick out a grey hair or two and lament that the full head of hair did not come up to the sample he had been shown, that so far from being worth the three half-crowns he had mentioned, it was useless to him. 'But as it's aff, and partly by my own fault, I'll gie a trifle, lass. I'll no be unjust, I'll gie half the money, though I may be a sair loser by the deal; but, ah! lass, why dinna ye suffer me attentively to examine the entire web afore I cut . . .?'

Another perfectly serious source of hair for wigs, which is still made use of, is combings. These are the hairs which come out naturally when they have finished their life cycle. The normal life of a hair is from three to seven years, though some illnesses cause hair to be shed prematurely. When long hair was fashionable, women made a point of saving the combings and keeping them in a special combing container on the dressing table. The resultant hair balls might be made up into a switch—if not used to stuff pin cushions—or simply sold to a hairdresser. The latter were accustomed also to receiving combings via pedlars who picked through heaps of domestic rubbish. Such was the value attached to human hair in almost any form.

No amount of tangles and foreign matter is any bar to the skilled posticheur turning lumps of combings into usable wigmaking hairs. The most unpromising material is transformed after the process of loosening, pulling bit by bit through a hackle, washing, disinfecting and turning. From the wigmaker's point of view almost the most important operation is the turning, which means getting all the root ends of a given quantity of hair together.

Hair used for wigmaking has to be made up so that it lies in the direction of growth. This is because hairs have overlapping scales, and run smooth from root to point but rough, as may be verified by finger and thumb, from point to root. If hair was sewn on a foundation with the roots and points mixed, the hairs would rub against each other and become tangled and difficult to comb. Fortunately for today's wigmakers, their raw material normally comes prepared for use by the hair merchants.

Sixteen

An outbreak of wigs

'An outbreak of wigs generally precedes ruin, the fall of kings, blood in the gutters . . . and someone on the point of saying "Let them eat cake".' This comes from an article by Siriol Hugh-Jones, published when the modern wigs craze was getting under way in 1962. She was presumably thinking of the glamorous Restoration wigs for men, which preceded a collapse of upper-class morals, and of all those towering female head-dresses at the end of the eighteenth century—just before the outbreak of the French Revolution.

At the time of writing, nine years after Miss Hugh-Jones's warning, it could be said that a state of ruin well describes the condition of many established institutions and forms of behaviour. An increased use of wigs has indeed been one of the precursors of change.

According to Jack Finger of the American journal *Salon Owner*, fashion wigs started coming back in 1958; they were inspired, he says, by a story in *Life* about the Carita sisters who were making wigs to match Givenchy's dresses. Proceeds from the sale of false hair in the United States have risen from about $4 million in 1960 to $500 million in 1970, in which year at least twenty firms were doing business amounting to over $1 million. When a Florida firm announced courses for hairdressers in the selling, fitting and maintenance of wigs, the response was almost embarrassing; some two thousand people wanted to attend one of the seminars.

Since 1960 the wig boom has been reflected in literally hundreds of articles and news stories in the Press on both sides of the Atlantic. In 1967, when numerous women and girls owned a cluster of seven or eight wigs of fashion, an able journalist called Polly Devlin wrote a piece in the London *Evening Standard* about how a wigged girl could imagine she had adopted a new personality. It was most entertaining. Having bought some wigs herself, as an experiment, Miss Devlin was able to report that men who had previously taken no notice of her grew suddenly attentive. 'It's like becoming a new person,' she said, 'but with a lovely escape clause—when you want to go back to being you, whip it off.' Miss Devlin suggested that the purchase of a few wigs might serve to cheer husbands and wives who had grown bored with each other.

In the spring of 1966 the London *Daily Express* had a write-up of a wig known as the Smoochy which was 'specially designed for the not-so-pretty girl'. It was silver-grey and covered half the face, including one eye. It was so glamorous, said the *Express* reporter, that any slight plainness still showing did not matter.

Items in the Press about women's wigs—all of which were concerned with fashion, by the way, rather than hiding scalp defects—became gradually outnumbered by items about male wigs to hide male loss of hair. It was clearly the assumption that the public was still able to feel a *frisson* of horror on reading of necessity wigs which for one reason or another let their wearers down.

In 1966 several papers carried a story about a shopkeeper, aged fifty-six, of Harlow in Essex, whose wig shrank after being tinted by a local barber, at the latter's suggestion. He sued, contending that not being able to wear his wig added twenty years to his apparent age. When he placed it on his head in court, the judge agreed that it could not be worn without embarrassment and awarded him 89 guineas (about $270) damages. The barber had this to say: 'It was a shocking fit in the first place and the carroty brown colour was ridiculous. I thought it looked better after my treatment.'

Another well reported incident concerned a Basingstoke

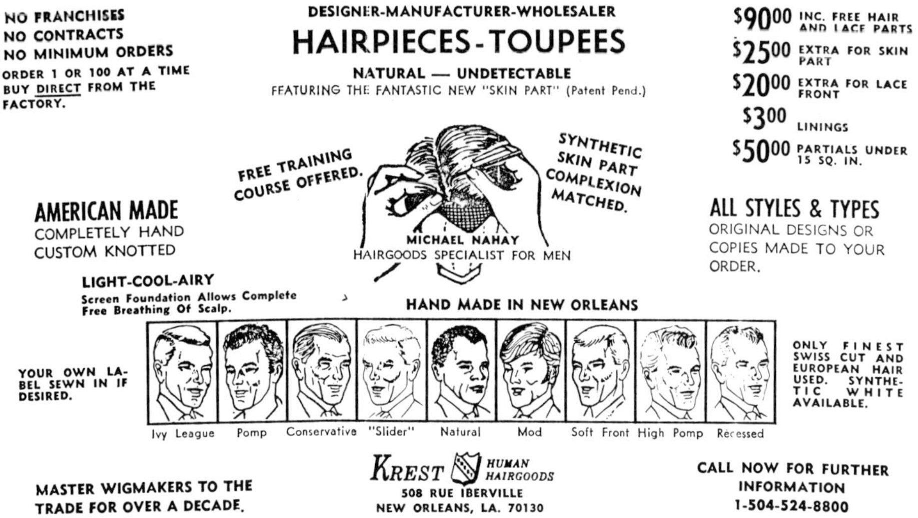

American trade advertisement for men's wigs

burglar who was readily traced by the police as a result of losing his partial wig in a scuffle at the scene of a burglary. He had invested in a very high-grade hairpiece (price £180, about $570) which the wigmaker had stamped with a six-figure serial number. It was said that he wept as he stood in the dock with his bald head bowed.

By 1967 some of the men with bald patches were beginning to wish that toupees were less exacting to wear. A Londoner who bought one but felt awkward in it, wrote to the *Evening Standard*: 'What about bringing back the fashion of wigs for men? There must be plenty who would welcome the idea. A toupet doesn't do much for a man . . . but a Charles II wig! That would be something.'

Later in 1967 Britain's Woolworth's began selling wigs from £2 (about $6) each. They had generous fringes and were usable by both men and women. By 1968 the stores were selling at 4s (about 50c) a suction base for wig holders;

it held them steady during combing.

Wide publicity attended the opening of Harrods' wig counter in 1969: false hair had arrived at London's most conservative store. Members of the Press were invited to watch the wigmaker fitting a volunteer demonstrator, a ware-houseman whose hair line had entirely disappeared. They noted that the way to find out where the hair used to be was to ask him to frown: the wigmaker set to work just above the point where the wrinkles stopped.

Most of the newspapers have given it out that twenty in every hundred men in Britain are to some extent bald; the figures are said to be similar in the United States, where the Society of Trichologists has predicted that the incidence of hair loss among men will gradually increase. Needless to say, these facts of life are less noticeable than they used to be to the casual observer. The *Sun* reported in 1970 that, thanks to the availability of wigs, 'Baldheads are vanishing in Britain at the rate of 100,000 a year—ten times faster than ten years ago'. An article in the London *Daily Telegraph Magazine* pointed out that the lack of an effective cure for baldness had left the way clear for 'a high pressure sales campaign which concentrates on the sex appeal and virility angles'.

Unlike women buying their fashion wigs, men may need clever salesmanship, apparently, if they are to be hooked. Robust-looking salesmen—they are often part-timers—

Cheap wigs of synthetic fibre from Hong Kong, *c.* 1970. Left, the Mia Farrow; right, the Vanda. Note how the hair line is covered. Both wigs weigh about four ounces knock on carefully selected doors in the evening or at the weekend. Almost invariably these travellers are bald. The reason for this was succinctly explained to a British reporter who followed up one of the first of the discreet advertisements for sales representatives with thinning hair. 'The job is selling wigs,' said the firm's spokesman, 'and it's very useful if, after half an hour's chat with a possible client, our men can clinch what they've been saying by removing a wig which the other man had taken for natural hair.'

In the United States it was estimated early in 1970 that a million and a half American men permanently wore full or partial wigs. Mr Mark Lorick, a leading supplier of ready-to-wear wigs and proprietor of two 'wig huts' at Richmond, Virginia, told a reporter: 'We feel the hair goods business is only just getting started. The boom is yet to come.' The first trade journal in English devoted entirely to wigs was launched at Port Lavaco, Texas, in July 1970. Here is a typical extract, concerning an idea for women's wigs: 'The two-in-one has the conventional wiglet base plus fourteen inserts, seven in one color, seven in another color or in an assortment of colors. It eliminates the normal frosting and streaking procedures. The insertion is so simple that a woman can do it herself.'

It has been estimated that 80 per cent of all the wigs sold in Britain are imported ready-made from Hong Kong. In the United States the suppliers of wigs put even greater reliance on the cheap labour of Far Eastern countries—Korea as well as Hong Kong. In March 1970 Britain's *Sunday Mirror* made a talking point by suggesting that some of the cheapest synthetic wigs from Hong Kong were dangerously inflammable compared with the human hair product. But hairdressers have been able to shrug this off, observing that most hats would catch on fire, too, if a lighted match was put to them. A far more lurid newspaper story would be needed to make a dent in the progress of an industry already worth, in Britain, £15 million (about $45 million) a year.

Included in this figure is around £1 million ($3 million) spent annually by the State on supplying wigs free on the National Health Service to people whose doctors consider they need them. This fact was revealed in 1970 in answer to a question in Parliament. Each patient, it was stated, had to have two wigs. Human hair was always used for N.H.S. wigs, and the average cost was £33 (about $100) each. There was no intention of making a change. Moreover, the State would continue to pay for the periodic cleaning.

The first accounts of men using fashion wigs to conceal their own extra long hair came from the United States. It seems that a short-haired wig in the pocket can come in useful at places where the police are interrogating 'hippies'. This is a curious variation of the much more usual use for men's fashion wigs which is illustrated by this report of September 1970: 'More than 2,000 U.S. servicemen at the Phantom jet base at Alconbury, Hants [England], have been told they may wear hairpieces, false moustaches, beards and side whiskers to hide military hair cuts when off duty.'

A spokesman said there were few social occasions at which a military haircut was looked on with disfavour, but there was no reason why the men should not wear wigs if this would help them to be accepted by people outside the base. They would not be creating a precedent, he said: 'Men in George Washington's day, and Washington himself, wore wigs.'

Notes

1 *Analysis of Beauty.*
2 Quoted by Friedrich Nicolai, *Uber der Gebrauch der falschen Haar und Perruken*, 1801.
3 Charles Desplanques, *Barbiers, perruquiers, coiffeurs*, Paris, 1927.
4 R. Turner Wilcox, *The Mode in Hats and Headdress*, New York, 1948.
5 Contemporary description quoted by Louis Ducros, *French Society in the Eighteenth Century*, Bell, 1926.
6 Dr J. Doran, *Habits and Men*, Bently, 1855.
7 *Oxinden Letters*, 1647, quoted by C. W. and Phillis Cunnington in *English Costume in the 17th Century*, Faber, 1955.
8 Aphra Behn, *The Dutch Lover*, quoted by James Laver in *Clothes*, Burke, 1952.
9 Gladys Scott Thomson, *Life in a Noble Household 1641–1700*, Cape, 1937.
10 Ralph Edwards, *The Shorter Dictionary of English Furniture*, Country Life, 1964.
11 F. Nicolai, op. cit.
12 Quoted by C. W. and Phillis Cunnington in *English Costume in the 18th Century*, Faber, 1957.
13 James Stevens Cox, *Dictionary of Hairdressing and Wigmaking*, Hairdressers' Technical Council, 1966.
14 *Plocacosmos or The Whole Art of Hairdressing*, 1782.
15 C. W. and Phillis Cunnington, *English Costume in the 18th Century.*
16 Ibid.
17 Ibid.
18 Ibid.
19 James Stevens Cox, op. cit.
20 Lawrence Wright, *Clean and Decent*, Routledge & Kegan Paul, 1960.
21 James Derriman, *The Pageantry of the Law*, Eyre & Spottiswoode, 1955.
22 John Nevinson in an introduction to *The Exact Dress of the Head*, Costume Society, 1970.
23 F. Nicolai, op. cit.
24 L. Ducros, op. cit.
25 G. d'Eze, *Histoire de la coiffure des femmes en France*, Paris, 1886.

26 C. W. and Phillis Cunnington, *English Costume in the 18th Century.*
27 *Hairdressers' Weekly Journal*, 1887.
28 Edited by John Beresford, Routledge, 1927.
29 Phillis Cunnington and Catherine Lucas, *Occupational Costume in England*, A. & C. Black, 1967.
30 Leonard Everett Fisher, *The Wigmakers*, Colonial American Craftsmen, New York, 1965.
31 John Gloag, *A Short Dictionary of Furniture*, Allen & Unwin, 1969 edn.
32 Letter quoted by Jean Keyes, *Women's Hairstyles*, Methuen, 1967.
33 C. W. and Phillis Cunnington, *English Costume in the 18th Century.*
34 Ibid.
35 Ibid.
36 J. Stevens Cox, op. cit.
37 F. Nicolai, op. cit.
38 Robert Seymour and Alfred Crowquill, *Humorous Sketches*, 1834.
39 J. Stevens Cox, op. cit.
40 Part of a poem, *c.* 1870, anon., quoted by James Laver, op. cit.
41 James Laver, op. cit.
42 James Derriman, op. cit.
43 Croake James, *Curiosities of the Law and Lawyers*, Low, 1891.
44 James Derriman, op. cit.
45 C. W. and Phillis Cunnington, *English Costume in the 17th Century.*

Index

Page numbers in italics denote illustrations

C

D

E

F

I

J

K

L

M

N

O

P

Q

R

S

Y